Praise for *Truth Doesn't Have a Side*

If you want to understand Dr. Bennet Omalu, don't look at the acronyms that come after his name or read the papers he's authored; listen to his laugh. It's the laugh of someone who possesses the freedom that can only come when you know that you are doing *exactly* what you were destined to do.

Will Smith

The name Bennet Omalu is one that many people may not be familiar with. But if you are a current or former athlete, a wife or a significant other of an athlete, or a parent of an athlete who competes or has competed in a contact sport that could produce concussions, his is a name you *should* know. His discovery of CTE gave a name to a cause of a neurological condition that many former athletes suffered from later in life. For many former football players like me, Dr. Omalu is our hero because he was that one person astute and bold enough to dig deeper in his neuropathology research to discover the cause of neurological ailments that may have affected countless former athletes long after the cheering stopped.

Harry Carson, New York Giants (1976–1988), and a member of the Professional Football Hall of Fame, class of 2006

Truth Doesn't Have a Side is a critically important book. If you care about your brain or the brains of those you love, please read it.

Daniel G. Amen, MD, author of *Memory Rescue*

Dr. Bennet Omalu's tireless pursuit of the truth is inspiring, and being able to relive his journey alongside him makes it all the more incredible. The world is a better place with doctors like Bennet Omalu in it.

Giannina Scott, actress and producer

The world craves elite examples of courage from selfless crusaders who genuinely care first about the needs of others. Dr. Omalu is that man, and his story will inspire you and challenge the sleeping hero in each of us!

Ben Utecht, musician, former NFL player, and author
of *Counting the Days While My Mind Slips Away*

Truth Doesn't Have a Side is a provocative, passionate, and enlightening discussion of football, forensic science, and religious faith. Dr. Bennet Omalu's research has focused much-needed attention on sports-related brain injuries. Whether readers agree or disagree with Dr. Omalu's dramatic conclusions, they will find his life story fascinating, highly informative, and truly remarkable.

Dr. Cyril Wecht, forensic pathologist and medicolegal
consultant; past president, American Academy of Forensic
Sciences and American College of Legal Medicine

Truth Doesn't Have a Side tells the remarkable story of Dr. Bennet Omalu's journey of perseverance in an imperfect world and his reliance on the absolute faithfulness of God. It is the story of what it means to be a disciple of Jesus.

Father Carmen D'Amico, pastor of Miraculous
Medal Parish, Meadow Lands, Pennsylvania

TRUTH
DOESN'T HAVE A SIDE

TRUTH
DOESN'T HAVE A SIDE

My Alarming Discovery
about the Danger
of Contact Sports

DR. BENNET OMALU

with Mark Tabb

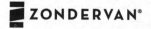

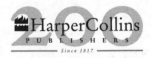

To my wife, Prema,
my daughter, Ashly, and my son, Mark—
you are all I live for.
I love you.

Contents

Foreword

I used to love football. Some of my fondest memories came watching my oldest son, Trey, stretch for the pylon beneath Friday Night Lights. He was a wide receiver; I was a proud dad doing my best to keep from running onto that field myself. That's the nice thing about being a spectator: it's easy, when you're watching from the safety of the sidelines. One step forward, though, and the game—like life—has a way of hitting you in the mouth. But shock can be good for the system. Challenge yourself, and you'll likely be surprised at what you learn. And what did I learn from playing the role of a Nigerian-born forensic pathologist in *Concussion*? I learned what it means to be American.

If you want to understand Dr. Bennet Omalu, don't look at the acronyms that come after his name or read the papers he's authored; listen to his laugh. It's the laugh of someone who possesses the freedom that can only come when you know that you are doing *exactly* what you were destined to do. It was that laugh—not the accent, the body language, or the medical jargon—that I knew I had to capture if I hoped to do justice to Dr. Omalu and his legacy. And while many will cite his discovery of CTE as his lasting contribution, I choose to point to his fearlessness in the face of derision, exile, and skepticism. That courage is what is quintessentially American about Dr. Omalu: when everyone thought him a kook, a fraud, or worse, he persevered and held fast to what he scientifically knew to be true, at great personal and professional risk. Life punched him in the mouth, but he kept fighting. He endured that initial shock in order to bring closure to the grieving families of so many whose deaths would have otherwise gone ignored or misdiagnosed.

I still love football. Ironically, I have Dr. Omalu to thank for that.

While Trey wore a helmet and pads and Dr. Omalu wears a white coat, they have something in common: day after day, they fought, yard by yard, to attain something they knew they deserved—a touchdown, or the truth. And what's more American than that?

Thank you, Dr. Omalu, for reminding me why I love this game, and this country.

Will Smith

God Did Not Intend for Human Beings to Play Football

Wherever I go, people ask me one question more than any other: "Dr. Omalu, is it safe for my child to play football?" The answer is simple. "No. It is not." I believe God did not make human beings to play football, especially children. Full-contact football is not safe for children, nor do I believe football can be made safe for adults. Of course, an adult can weigh the risks and rewards of playing and make the decision for himself or herself. Children cannot do so, for their brain, mind, intellect, intuition, and understanding are not yet fully developed. As a society, we recognize this fact and do not allow children to smoke cigarettes, drink alcohol, or engage in other high-risk activities. We do this to protect children from themselves until they have the maturity to weigh the risks and rewards and make an informed decision for themselves. That is why I believe no one under the age of eighteen should be allowed to play football. Period.

Should adults play? I do not think so, but that is their decision. However, before any adult steps onto a football field, they need to understand that nothing protects the human brain from the force of impact experienced in full-contact sports. God did not design us for such impact. He did so for other animals. The woodpecker has a built-in shock absorber to protect its brain as it bangs into the side of a tree.

Woodpeckers can play football safely. Humans cannot—not even with the latest state-of-the-art equipment. Helmets protect the skin and the skull and keep the skull from fracturing, but no helmet can ever provide complete cushioning for the brain.

Why does this matter? The brain, unlike most other organs that make up the human body, does not have the capacity to cure itself. Broken legs heal; neurons do not. When brain cells are damaged or die in both concussive and sub-concussive hits, they are gone. That is why I believe football can never be made safe, at least not in anything approaching the form of the game today.

• • • •

The next question I am asked is, "Why are you so against football? Why do you hate the game?" I plead innocence. I do not hate football. I have nothing against the game itself. My wife, Prema, grew up in Kenya and never saw an American football game until she moved to this country in 2001. Almost immediately she was captivated by the beauty and elegance of the game. I must admit, it is a beautiful game, albeit a violent beauty. When I see the sport through her eyes, I can see why so many millions love the game. It is a wonder to behold when it is played at a high level.

But I did not learn the game by watching it on the field or on television. My introduction to football came when one of the greatest players to ever play the game came to me, hoping I might be able to find the answer to why he died far too young and why he suffered so much torment the last years of his life. People thought he had lost his mind because he had lost his memory and frequently could not remember his way home. Mike also battled depression and other mood disorders. By the time I met Mike, he was addicted to drugs, had lost his intelligence, and could not hold his thought or engage in complex reasoning. In the end, he was bankrupt and homeless.

When Mike Webster died, people used respectful terms to describe his playing career, yet there was an underlying, almost a mocking tone that questioned why he made so many poor choices that ruined his life after he retired from football. I heard these people describe his life as tragic and a waste. Then I met Mike Webster on the autopsy table. When I met him, I knew I had to find the answers for the problems that plagued him. This was my calling, my duty as a fellow human being made in the image of God.

My search for answers and justice for Mike Webster introduced me to the game of football. Before I ever watched a single play on the field, I observed the toll the game takes on the human body, especially the brain. Mike Webster suffered from a completely preventable brain malady called Chronic Traumatic Encephalopathy, or CTE. I say preventable because if Mike Webster had never played football, he almost certainly would still be alive today, and the two of us would never have had reason to meet.

So what do I have against football? Why do I hate the game? I do not hate it, but I hate the toll it takes on those who play it. Does that mean I am against football? No, not if you mean I am against adults exercising their God-given right to choose to play football. If someone knows the risks and chooses to play, God bless them. However, I would never play, and I would never allow my children to play, and I encourage my friends not to let their children play. My outlook might be very different if Mike Webster had been an anomaly, but he was not. I believe there is a very good chance that every person who plays (or has played or will play) in the NFL will suffer from some degree of CTE. Not everyone will suffer to the degree Mike Webster did, but some will be worse.

• • • •

The next question people ask is not really a question. It is more an accusation, hurled at me in anger. "Who are you, an outsider, an African—not even an African *American*—to cast such a cloud over America's most popular sport?" When I first published my findings on the impact of football on the human brain, I was attacked. The National Football League accused me of falsifying my research. Some claimed I practiced voodoo, not medicine. The onslaught of attacks against me and my character grew so intense that I eventually lost my job, my dream home, and nearly everything I had worked so hard to achieve. Even today, my work is marginalized, and my role in bringing football's "brain crisis" to light has been dismissed.

"Who are you?" is the underlying question, the accusation, that follows me wherever I go. Does it follow me because of the color of my skin or because of the nation of my birth? Perhaps. But whatever the reason, I welcome the question. Who am I indeed? I've asked the question myself. Why was I the one who first discovered CTE in the brain of an American football player? Why was I the one who pulled back the curtain on the NFL's dirty little secret and forced it to deal with questions it sought to hide for many years?

Believe me, my life would have been much simpler if I had never met Mike Webster. I was living the American dream and counting my blessings every day to have such a wonderful life. I might have had to wrestle with the question of whether or not a child should be allowed to play football, but that would have been a personal decision for my wife and me in regard to our son and daughter. No one else would have cared about my opinion on the question, nor would I have felt qualified to give one.

But all that changed the day I met Mike Webster. It changed again when movie director Peter Landesman entered my life, and even more when Will Smith came to see me as he prepared to play me in the movie *Concussion*. Now I am the man people want to ask whether or not their children should play football. Why do they ask me? Who am I to answer such a question? That is why I am writing this book.

I never sought this life. God placed me here. I believe all that brought me to this place came as a direct result of the hand of God leading and directing my life. Who am I that the One who created the cosmos would bother with one so small? The answer is much larger than football.

Chapter One

My Father's Son

My father grew up an orphan. His father was a fisherman from the Igbo tribe in southern Nigeria. One day, my father's father drowned for no known reason. At least that's what his wife was told. They could not tell her how he died, and his body was never recovered. She never believed he drowned. My grandmother was convinced her husband had been murdered, since the circumstances surrounding his death were very suspicious with so many unanswered questions, but no one listened to her. No one investigated. "He drowned," she was told. "You must accept it and move on." She could not accept it. She needed answers, but none ever came. Finally she became so angry and frustrated that she just ran away, leaving behind my three-year-old father and his one-and-a-half-year-old sister, Nwanedo, to fend for themselves. My grandmother eventually reentered my father's life, but not for decades.

With no one to care for them, my father and his little sister ended up wandering the streets of the town of Enugwu-Ukwu, begging for food. Ironically, my father's father gave him a name that expressed optimism and hope for the future. In the Igbo tribal culture, as in many parts of the world, names are given because of their meanings. A name conveys a blessing to the one who hears it. My father's name was Amaechi, which means, "I may be down today, but no one knows what tomorrow may bring!"

My grandfather's prayer was answered, for, as divine providence would have it, the local Roman Catholic priest, a missionary, noticed my father and his sister and took them in. He asked one of the leaders of the local church to take care of my father as a foster child, while another family took in his sister. Because of the kindness of the priest, my father began attending church and eventually became a Christian. My father's new family allowed him to go to the local school run by the Catholic missionaries, probably at the insistence of the priest who found him on the street. My aunt was not so lucky. Her family did not send her to school, nor did they treat her well. Later in life, she ended up financially dependent on my father for her most basic needs.

Even with the privilege of pursuing an education, life was very hard for my father. His foster family never considered him a son. They treated him more like a servant, which was not uncommon for orphans in the 1920s in Nigeria. Every day, my father worked from morning until night, doing chores, helping cook the meals and clean the house, and attending to all the needs of the master's children—even though my father was a child himself. But that was not all. When I was old enough to understand, my father showed me the scars on his face and body where he had been physically abused by his foster parents and their children. He also experienced a great deal of emotional abuse. Many days, he ran out the door to school hungry because there wasn't enough food left for him after everyone else in the family ate. A firm slap on the face or a hard knock on the head awaited him every time he did what children do—like spilling water accidentally on the floor.

Even with the hardships, my father considered himself very blessed because he had the opportunity to go to school. Each day, he had to take care of the master's children and see them off to school before getting himself cleaned up and ready for class. But he got to go to school. Very early on, my father realized that education gave him his only opportunity to become somebody and improve his lot in life. He worked very hard in his studies and graduated from high school. However, he could not afford college. Instead, he found a job as the personal assistant to the local colonial administrator who worked in the Ministry of Mines and

Power. Up until 1960, Nigeria was a colony of Britain. My father's new boss was English.

With the new job, my father became his own man who made a good living and earned his own income. His boss noticed my father's exceptional attitude toward work. No matter how tedious or demanding the work, my father never complained. For him, work was a blessing, for now he was free from his past abuse and no longer had to suffer in silence just to stay alive. My father loyally served his boss, so much so that when his boss eventually retired and moved back to England, he asked my father, "What can I do for you to repay you for your faithful service to me?"

My father gave the question a lot of deep thought. He might have asked for some tangible material things, like the man's car he was leaving behind or some of his belongings he could not take to England. Instead, my father went back to the revelation he had at the missionary school: Through education you can become anyone you want to be. A car will wear out and have to be replaced, but an education sticks with you for the rest of your life and opens doors that will not open any other way. "Can you help me go to college?" my father asked his departing boss. Like father, like son, I grew up to develop the same faith in education. I saw education as an empowering tool that would enable me to become the man I was born to be. I sought after education with all my might.

The man was very impressed with my father's humble request. "Of course," he said. True to his word, the man secured a scholarship for my father to study mining engineering at the Camborne School of Mines in Penryn, Cornwall, England. He also gave my dad some of his material things he could not take back to England.

Prior to leaving for England for college, my father met a woman named Chiwude and wanted to marry her. Chiwude means "God provides the ink with which we write our lives." She also had an English name, Caroline. When my father went to Caroline's father and asked for her hand in marriage, her father refused. "My first daughter will not marry an orphan," he insisted. Giving up on that relationship, my father met another woman, and the two were soon engaged. However, the relationship did not work out, and they broke off the engagement. My father was single and alone when he moved to England not long after the end of the Second World War.

When my father arrived in Cornwall, he rented a room in the home of a childless couple who had been trying to have a baby for years without success. Miraculously, a few months after my father moved in, the couple conceived a child. They were overjoyed, but my father had to find a new place to stay, as his room became the baby's room. My father moved in with another childless couple, who also conceived a few months after his arrival. Word spread. Many childless couples wanted my father to move in with them. They nicknamed him "the Black Cat"—only this black cat brought good luck.

His living conditions aside, my father devoted all his energy to his studies. Four years after arriving in England, this former street child, the once abused orphan, graduated with a degree in mining engineering. For a child of the street to even find a family was and still is remarkable. For that child to graduate from high school was so unusual as to be thought of as impossible. Yet, as my father's name testifies, you never know what tomorrow may bring. Tomorrow brought my father a college degree from an English university. I struggle to find words to convey to you the emotions this stirs inside of me. My father was abandoned at the age of three, yet when he moved back to Nigeria from England with his degree in hand, he ascended to a position of great authority and respect. Rather than serve as someone's assistant, my father became his own boss at the Ministry of Mines and Power and the boss of many other men. Only God could bring about such a tomorrow.

During my father's time in England, he traveled back to Nigeria once to try to convince Caroline's father to give him a chance. Her father refused to change his mind. After returning to Nigeria for good, my father met another woman and was soon engaged. Once again, the relationship fell apart. Heartbroken, my father poured his energy into his work, earning high praise for his skills and work ethic.

A few years later, my father was told Caroline now found herself in a different situation. Her father had died suddenly from a ruptured appendix. After his death, Caroline had to drop out of school and go to work to support her brothers and sisters. The boys in the family stayed in school because, at the time, it was a better investment to educate boys rather than girls. Boys had more opportunities open to them. Caroline opened a small, street-side dress shop but the business struggled. She found herself alone, poor, and broken.

My father went to Caroline and once again asked her to marry him. Rather than being a poor, abused orphan, my father was now a graduate of an English college, a civil servant with a good job and a bright future. With her father no longer around to object, Caroline said yes to his proposal, and the two were married in 1958 and remained married for fifty-six years until my father's death in 2014.

Given the way my father pursued my mother, it might be easy to assume that he had fallen so deeply in love with her that he could not rest until he had her. Yet I vividly remember my father telling me, "Bennet, never marry because you have fallen in love. Never come to me and tell me that you are getting married because you are so much in love that you cannot live without this woman. If you fall in love, then you can fall out of love, for it is often nothing but infatuation, a type of foolish love." He went on to tell me that when you love a woman, it is a conscious decision to love, adore, and accept her for who she is. When you truly love, you do whatever is within your means to bring out the woman she is and the woman she was born to be. You seek to make her happy. "Love should not control you," he told me. "Rather, you control it. It is a rational decision you make to love sacrificially, even when it is demanding and difficult and painful." I know this is how my parents were able to have a strong marriage for fifty-six years. For a man who grew up as an orphan, a mistreated foster child, he had a great deal of insight into what it means to truly love someone.

My mother and father settled into a middle-class lifestyle and soon started a family. Two years after my mother and father married, Britain granted Nigeria her independence. My father continued in his same position with the Ministry of Mines and Power. He worked in several towns across Nigeria but spent most of his time in the northern city of Jos. Over the next eight years, he and my mother had five children. My father, who now went by the English name John, believed that the emerging English culture and economic system of the West would eventually dominate globally. Therefore, he thought it socially and economically strategic for each of his children to have an English name. He named my five oldest siblings Theodore, Winnifred, Henrietta, Ignatius, and Edwin; my only younger sister, Mirian. But my parents also wanted to bestow a blessing upon their children and give them names that were, in essence, a prayer over each of them. They named my oldest brother Onyekwelu, which means, "Who believed I would become somebody in life?" Winnifred they named Chinyelu—"This is God's gift to me." Henrietta is Uchenna—"This is the will of God." Ignatius is Ikemefuna— "May my strength not be taken from me." Edwin is Chizoba—"May God save and protect us." And finally, Mirian is Ekenedilichukwu—"To God be all the glory and thanks."

My parents had a good life, and it might have continued forever if not for events they could not control. Most of the boundaries in the countries of Africa have nothing to do with traditional tribal areas. Nor do they really have anything to do with the way people historically self-identified. The vast majority of the boundaries on the continent were created by the European powers that colonized them. (Ethiopia is the biggest exception, as it was the only African nation that fought back successfully and was never colonized.) As a result, people of different— and sometimes warring—tribes and religions found themselves thrown together because of treaties negotiated between governments thousands of miles away that took nothing into consideration except lines on a map.

In Nigeria, the arbitrary boundaries established by Great Britain left the nation with a predominantly Muslim population made up of the Hausa people in the north and a predominantly Christian population in the south primarily composed of the Yoruba and Igbo people. During the colonial era, tensions between the north and south did not boil over into violence, because both still saw themselves as separate. Britain treated each area differently from the other. However, once the English left, the two very different parts of the country were thrown together into one. The newly independent nation got off to a rocky start. In May 1966, General Aguiyi-Ironsi, an Igbo general in the Nigerian army, took over the government after a foiled coup. A few months later, Muslims from the north launched a countercoup and killed General Aguiyi-Ironsi.

As tensions grew, my father moved his family four hundred miles south to the predominantly Igbo town of Enugwu-Ukwu. Jos was in the Muslim north. My father continued working in Jos and came home to the family as often as he could. At this time, my parents had their fifth child, Chizoba, which means "May God save and protect us," a prayer for our family, which needed protection—as did all the Igbo people. Fearing they would be marginalized in the government, the southern tribes of Nigeria, led by the Igbos, declared their own independence on May 30, 1967. They created a new nation in southeast and southwest Nigeria called Biafra, which was Christian. Civil war with the north and west (which were predominately Muslim and mixed Muslim-Christian, respectively) broke out almost immediately.

When war broke out, my father was in Jos. It was the worst place he could have been. The war was not fought on faraway battlefields. Nigerian government forces and northern Muslim tribes started slaughtering Igbos wherever they found them in the north. Since Jos had a large Igbo population, the slaughter was fierce there. My father immediately went into hiding, but he knew he could not hide forever. He had to get to the south, but he could not just jump on a train with a ticket to Biafra. The moment he showed himself in public, he was in danger of death. He did not know what to do.

Thankfully, God sent an angel to carry my father home. Even though the British had officially pulled out of the country, many still remained in important jobs. My father worked alongside an expatriate British man, and the two had become friends. As the slaughter started, his British friend told my father, "I will get you home." The friend had my father lie down in the back of his Land Rover and covered him with a blanket, clothes, and even luggage. He made sure there was a small opening to give my father air to breathe. With no other option, my father agreed to his friend's plan, while also surrendering himself to the will of Almighty God. When he climbed into the back of the Land Rover, my father prepared himself for the very real possibility that he would not get out alive.

Military checkpoints were set up all along the roads between Jos and Biafra. My father's friend had not driven far before he came to the first checkpoint. The tribesmen manning it carried automatic rifles, spears, bows and arrows, and machetes. They motioned for my father's friend to pull over, but when they saw that he was white, they waved him on without searching his car. The same thing happened at the next checkpoint—and the next and the next.

About the time my father felt like he could relax, the car stopped again. Angry voices barked out orders. Then my father heard a key go into the trunk lock. He held his breath. The back hatch of the Land Rover opened. More angry voices chattered away. The luggage lying on top of my father moved back and forth. If the angry person conducting the search were to dig down a little deeper, my father would be found. *O God, protect me. Take me home to my family*, my father prayed as he tried to calm his heart and not move a muscle. Then, without warning, the hatch slammed shut and the car was back on its way down the road.

They encountered a few more checkpoints. One or two other times, people looked into the back of the Land Rover, but only for a moment. No one dug around. No one really searched the vehicle because the driver was a white Englishman. I guess the tribesmen from the north assumed that no white man would risk his life for an Igbo.

Eventually, my father's friend drove through the final checkpoint and entered Biafra. He went a little farther into the country and stopped at a major crossroad called Ninth Mile Junction, about nine miles outside of Enugu. My father climbed out of the back of the vehicle and embraced his friend. "You saved my life. I will never forget what you did for me and my family," my father said.

"I will write to you to make sure you are okay," his friend replied. Their good-bye had to be fast. Even though my father was near home, he was not completely safe. He caught a bus at the crossroad and went home.

The British friend saved my father's life, but my family was not safe in Enugwu-Ukwu. Nigerian armed forces invaded the seceded Biafra. Because Enugwu-Ukwu was a major town in Biafra, it came under attack. My father led our family as they fled south and west as refugees to the town of Nnokwa. The war intensified. Nigerian forces encircled Biafra and set up a blockade. No food or aid could come in or out. Hunger and starvation became weapons of war. Biafran people, most of whom were Igbo, began to suffer from malnutrition and starve to death. Every day, hundreds and thousands of men, women, children, and babies died of hunger and disease. Of the more than two million casualties in Biafra during the war, nearly all were civilians.

Word of the crisis spread to the world. *Life* magazine featured two young Igbo children on its cover with the headline "Starving Children of Biafra War." Even today, when I see photos of the war, I weep. The United Nations responded by holding talks about the war, but that's all they did. They talked and talked, but nothing was done. Britain, the country that had ruled Nigeria for so long, did nothing to bring the two sides together. Instead, they supplied weapons to the northern Nigerian armed forces.

My family suffered through the war. Even though my father was a graduate of an English college and had faithfully served as a government civil servant for many years, when war broke out, he was just Igbo. Nothing he had done before mattered. My family moved in with relatives as refugees, losing everything my father had worked all his life to attain. At the refugee camp, my family, like nearly everyone else in Biafra, relied on food drops from the Red Cross and CARITAS, the international Catholic relief agency, to survive. At first, trucks were able to get through and deliver the food, coming up from Port Harcourt, Biafra's primary link to the outside world. However, on May 19, 1968, Port Harcourt fell to the Nigerian forces. After that, food had to be dropped out of airplanes and delivered via parachutes to the refugee camps.

The Nigerian armed forces increased the severity of their attacks. Not only did the Nigerian air force bomb military targets, but they also bombed agricultural areas and other places where civilians lived. Biafran officials pleaded with the world to act, but no one did. For the people of Biafra, including the Igbo tribe, the war went from bad to worse.

And in the midst of the worst part of the civil war, my mother discovered she was pregnant with her sixth child. Me.

Chapter Two

Child of War

W hen I run into people these days at the airport or grocery store or gym, wherever I go, many people recognize me. They have seen me on the news or in the PBS documentary *League of Denial* or in photos with Will Smith connected to the movie *Concussion*, where Will played me. Almost every time someone recognizes me, they tell me how much they admire me. "Oh my gosh," they say to me, "you are a hero to me for what you have done." Many young ones tell me they want to be like me when they get older. Most want to take a selfie with me.

I smile and pose for the photograph and thank them for their kind words, but I do not feel I belong on the pedestal on which they have placed me. They only see the Bennet Omalu of today. In their eyes, I am a success, a polished, finished product. What bothers me after the photos are taken and the admirers walk away is that they do not know the whole story. Much of my life has been filled with struggles and failures, weakness and doubt. Yet these difficulties, my Calvary, made me the man I am today and give substance to my life's work. I may be a success today, not because of where I am in life or what I have done, but because of where I began and the path I have traveled. Our journeys define us, and my journey was rocky from the start.

. . . .

Because the Nigerian army and naval blockade of Biafra kept most supplies from getting through to the south during the civil war in which I was born, food was very, very scarce when my mother discovered she was pregnant. Why my parents chose to conceive me at this time I will never know. The fact that I survived long enough to be born is a miracle.

Another miracle occurred the week of my birth. When my mother went into labor with me, my father was delayed at work at his Biafran government post. She went to the refugee hospital and tried to get word to my father to join her there. Not long after she arrived at the hospital, the air-raid sirens sounded. Nigerian war planes flew in low overhead and dropped bombs on the town of Nnokwa, where we lived as refugees. The planes arrived just as my father walked out into the street from where he had been posted by the government of Biafra. He took off running as bombs exploded all around him. An explosion knocked him to the ground. He tried to move but couldn't. Shrapnel filled his body. The air raid lasted only a few minutes. When the planes flew away, rescuers found my father's bleeding body. They assumed he was dead and were surprised when he let out a low groan. Since he showed signs of life, they took him to the closest hospital, which also happened to be the place where I had just been born. They took him to the emergency room, but no one expected him to live.

A refugee hospital is nothing like a typical American hospital. Few doctors work there, and those who do have to do everything. For me, this meant that the doctor who cared for my mother through her labor was the same doctor who wrapped my father's wounds with bandages, Dr. Ifeakandu. Coincidentally, the doctor's name is an Igbo word that means "life is the greatest gift of all." On the week of my birth, the full drama of life played out. In one room, my father lay dying, moribund; in the next, I lay crying, having just entered the world. Outside, the air-raid sirens blared, bombs exploded, and a war went on.

But here is the real miracle. A few days after he was hit with shrapnel, my father turned a corner and began to recover. The doctor and staff had told my mother to prepare for his death. Instead he survived and went on to a complete recovery.

When I was several weeks old, my father was finally well enough to sit up and see me. They carried me into his room and placed me in his arms. My father looked at me and said, "Your name will be Bennet, from the French word *benoit*—to bless. You, my son, are a blessing to me and will be a blessing." My parents also gave me the middle name Ifeakandu, after the doctor who took care of my father, my mother, and me. My last name, Omalu, is actually a shortened version of our full family name, Onyemalukwube, which means "If you know, come forth and speak." This means my full name is "A blessing . . . Life is the greatest gift of all . . . If you know, come forth and speak." My parents bestowed this name upon me, but I believe it was God who chose it. Even though no one could have known it on the day my father held me and named me, my name set the course for my entire life and has defined the man whom God created me to be.

· · · ·

The war ended when I was two years old. After three years of war, the Igbo people surrendered and Biafra was no more. Between two and four million Igbos died in the war. Once the war ended, the country of Nigeria tried to act like it had never happened. The name Biafra was erased from the history books, and Nigeria came back together as one. No one complained, because most people wanted to put the scars and pain of the war behind them.

To speed the recovery process, the Nigerian government gave £20, or about $48, to every Biafran family that had a bank account before the war. (Because Nigeria had been an English colony, its monetary system was based on the British model until 1973.) We were supposed to start over with this money. Not mentioned was the fact that any money anyone had in the bank prior to the war was now the property of the government, even if it totaled £100,000. All of our family's savings were wiped out, as were the savings of all the Igbo people. We were now the poorest people in a poor country, labeled losers forever. But at least our family had the £20 with which to start over.

The Nigerian government rehired my father, although in a diminished position. He gladly took the job. Like everyone else in our country, he wanted to move on from the war and rebuild a life for his family. But life was now different, even at work. All the people my father had once supervised were now his superiors. He lost his years of service and other benefits he'd accumulated over the years. However, he felt blessed just to have a job. He and my mother tried to just get on with life. They had another child, my sister Mirian, whose Igbo name, Ekenedilichukwu, means "To God be all the glory and thanks."

Although I have no memory of the war or the bombings or the food shortages, the experience changed my life forever. I suffered some war-related malnutrition during my first two years of life. My mother told me that I did not taste meat or fresh produce until after the war was over. When I had my first taste of meat, I spat it out with disgust. I've since made up for that. My body never caught up to where I should have been in terms of growth. I was always the smallest of all the children in my family, standing at five feet seven inches tall as an adult. Even my baby sister passed me sizewise before I was even ten years old.

My small stature bothered me very much. It didn't help that my brothers and sisters made fun of me, as brothers and sisters will always do. "Bennet is lazy," they said because I didn't like manual labor. "Bennet is weak," they said because I was so small. "Bennet never works; he just wants to study his books and play his games. What is wrong with you?" they said. They laughed at me all the time.

One afternoon, I'd had enough. My mother stood in the kitchen dishing out lunch for me and my brothers and sisters. As always, I was right there with her. Growing up, I never left my mother's side. On this day, I looked up at her and asked a question that had bothered me for some time. "Mommy," as I fondly called her, "why am I the shortest in the family?" By this time, my little sister Mirian was nearly as tall as me.

My mother quietly set down the dishing spoon. She bent down and looked me right in the eyes. "Benc," she called me, as everyone in the family did, "God is the One who makes you tall or short. Your height is beyond your control. But it is within your control as to what you choose to make of yourself. You can become the tallest man in the world in whatever you choose to do with your life." She paused for a moment, still looking directly into my eyes. Then she asked, "Do you understand what I just told you?"

"Yes, Mommy," I said.

My mother continued looking into my eyes. I could see the loving pain in her eyes. "Bene, do not worry that God made you short because if you work hard, you can become anything you wish, even the tallest man in the world in whatever you choose to do. Do you understand what I am telling you?" she asked a second time.

"Yes, Mommy, I understand," I said.

My mother stood up and went back to working on our lunch. I walked over to the cabinet and grabbed the dishes to set the table, just like I did for every meal. Now I did not feel so small. I believed my mother. Right then, I made up my mind that my physical size did not matter. I truly believed I could become anything I wanted to if I was willing to work hard enough to achieve it.

This new conviction did not bring about an immediate change in my behavior, however. I wasn't very motivated in school. Not only was I the smallest one in my class, but I was also the youngest. I started school when I was only three. My parents arranged for me to go to school with my brother Chizoba, not because I showed great academic ability, but because Chizoba was my first and greatest playmate. When he left for school, I cried uncontrollably until he returned home. Nothing my mother did could calm me down. Finally, she and my father asked the school principal if I could tag along to school for just a few days to help me get over my separation anxiety. Honestly, they didn't think I would stay more than a day or two. At the end of the week of my attending class, the principal had a question for my parents: "Bennet is outperforming many of the children in the class. How would you feel about letting him continue on in school?"

My parents were surprised by the request, but they didn't hesitate in saying yes. My father knew that education means power. He was more than happy to start his youngest son on the path as quickly as possible.

In spite of my strong beginning, my performance in school was nothing special. I did not bother to study, nor did I work hard at my studies. Sometimes I did, and my grades put me in the top 5 percent of my class. But then I grew bored and ignored my work. Then I found myself in the bottom 5 percent. Either way, it didn't matter to me. I carried on this same pattern all through primary school and into high school.

My grades may not have mattered to me, but they did to my oldest sister, Winny. She had already finished school and moved out of the house when she came home for Christmas one year. She saw my grades and laid into me. "Do you have two brains, Bennet?" she asked.

"What do you mean?"

"How can you go from the top of your class to the bottom and then back to the top?" she challenged me.

"I don't know," I replied.

"I know how. You are lazy, and if you keep this up, you will be a loser in life. Is that what you want—to be a loser?"

Her words made me very angry, and she knew it. I think that was her plan. She then added, "I tell you what. If you finish first in your class next term, I will give you fifty naira." That was the equivalent of fifty dollars. I was insulted, but I took her up on her offer. The next term, I finished first in my class and collected her money. After that, I never looked back. I spent hours upon hours reading, imagining things, and just thinking. I began to realize that knowledge is a powerful asset. I could not kick a soccer ball, which made my classmates laugh at me. But those same classmates were eager to come to me for help with a math problem or an English composition.

• • • •

Grades were something I found I could master if I applied myself, but I struggled socially. As a child I was very quiet and withdrawn. I did not have close friends outside of my family. Most of the time, I preferred to be home, either staying close to my mother or simply being by myself. I didn't feel like I was good at anything except my imagination. I discovered my imagination had no boundaries or limits. In the hours I spent by myself, I let my imagination take me all over the world. And my favorite place to go was America.

Growing up, my first exposure to America came through music. Since American music goes all over the world, this should come as no surprise. I liked what I heard, but I really identified with rhythm and blues and African-American singers. I couldn't get enough of Teddy Pendergrass, Tina Turner, Luther Vandross, Marvin Gaye, Dionne Warwick, Gladys Knight, Lionel Richie, Diana Ross, and Anita Baker. And of course, Whitney Houston and Michael Jackson. As odd as it may sound, I also listened to some country music from America, artists like Don Williams and Kenny Rogers. As I got older, I began to hear this new music called hip-hop. I liked it. Will Smith, Tupac, Jay Z, and Puff Daddy impressed me.

I liked American music, but what really grabbed me was the perfection the top American artists seemed to create. Occasionally I got to watch music videos on satellite television, and the perfection seemed even more pronounced. The creativity and the production value told me more about America than any newscast or history book. I was an emotional child, and I fell in love with this place, not because of any sociopolitical ideals but through the creativity and quality of their music. This perfection also seemed to know no bounds. Male or female, black or white, it didn't matter, they strove for perfection. I once saw Lionel Richie playing his piano and singing on television. I was in awe, for he seemed to personify the perfection God created us to attain. I promised myself that whatever I did in life, whatever job I someday had, I would strive for the same perfection. That is why I imagined myself in America.

Once while watching American television, I came across a game

Americans play, but it was unlike any game I had ever witnessed. The players dressed up like extraterrestrials with brightly colored helmets and bulging, protective gear under their clothes. They looked like broad-chested, big-headed, tiny-legged visitors from Mars. The game didn't make a lot of sense to me. The players purposefully ran into one another like trucks ramming each other on the highway. In soccer, you try to avoid running into the other players. If you hit someone on purpose, you get a yellow or red card. In this game, running into each other seemed to be the point. The name also confused me. Why did they call it "football," since people carried the ball in their hands and passed it with their hands to the other players? It was the oddest game I had ever witnessed.

Football aside, America was my favorite imaginary destination. For me, no place on earth came closer to heaven than the America I heard in music and watched on television and read about in books and magazines. I believed it to be the country that was closest to what God wants us to be as His sons and daughters, a place where you can be whatever you want, a place where you can be yourself. That's all I ever really wanted to be. Myself.

But I was not sure who I was. I often escaped to my imaginary world because the world in which I found myself as a boy was filled with disappointment and dissatisfaction. I struggled with low self-esteem. I had no reason to feel like this, because I grew up in a warm, loving family. Of course, my siblings made fun of me, but that's what siblings do. I gave it right back to them, just as much as they gave it to me.

However, in spite of the love I received from my family, I felt I was a loser in everything. Perhaps I had absorbed the label pressed upon the Igbo people after the war. In Nigeria, the Igbos were losers. I was Igbo. That made me a loser. I carried this feeling with me all the time. When I was around people, I felt like everyone looked down on me. My feelings of inadequacy caused me to pull more and more into myself, into the world where my imagination set me free. But I could not imagine my way out of the loneliness I felt.

The problem was I did not feel like I fit in anywhere, often not even at home. I had this driven home to me one Saturday morning when I was about thirteen. My father was a remarkable man. He reminded me of the traditional, cultured English gentleman who dressed so formally and so well, who spoke impeccable English, and who believed in proper English manners and etiquette. His years in England and working side by side with British nationals rubbed off on him in this way. Like any proper English gentleman, my father also had a beautiful garden in our home, and he expected his children to work in it.

Early one Saturday morning, I heard my father call out to my brother Chizoba, my sister Mirian, and me to get out of bed and come down to work the garden. My four older siblings no longer lived at home. Chizoba was the direct opposite of me. Energetic and sociable, he ran out and joined my father in the garden. Mirian fell right in behind him. Me, I rolled over and tried to ignore them. My mother came into my room. "Bene, get up. Your father is waiting for you. Time to get to work."

"I want to sleep," I said. I did want to sleep, but I also wanted to spend my day reading, alone.

My mother kept after me for a few minutes, without success. I should have obeyed her. Instead I laid in bed until my father, the proper English gentleman, burst into my room and in a less than genteel way made it very clear that I was to report to duty in the garden immediately or there would be serious consequences. I bounced out of bed, humiliated. When I went outside, my brother and sister glared at me. "It's about time," Mirian barked. Chizoba joined in chiding me. My father—he didn't say much. Instead he pointed to the worst part of the garden where the weeds were the thickest and the work was the hardest. "There," he said and pointed.

For the next few hours, I worked and sweated and became covered with dirt. When I was finally released from duty, I went back up to my room and shut the world out. I ran out onto the balcony off my room and sat down and cried. *Why can't people just leave me alone?* I wondered. Looking back, I understand why my father did what he did, and I also understand my brother's and sister's resentment toward me. I do not resent the fact that my father expected me to work. However, my real crisis came because I felt so ill at ease and so different from the rest of my family. The feeling washed over me and caused me to break into tears.

As I sat on my balcony, crying, I felt the Spirit of God speak to me. *Yes, you are different*, I felt the Spirit impress upon me, *but that is okay. You are who I made you to be. You are Bennet Ifeakandu Omalu, and there can never be another. There is only one you.* I thought about this truth for a long while. If I am the only me, I could not allow anyone else to define me or determine who I was or who I was to become. Jesus Himself said, "You are the light of the world. A city set on a mountain cannot be hidden. Nor do they light a lamp and then put it under a bushel basket; it is set on a lampstand, where it gives light to all in the house. Just so, your light must shine before others, that they may see your good deeds and glorify your heavenly Father"[1] These words came to my mind as the sky grew dark above me and the stars began to shine. God had made me who I was, and He made me and called me to let His light shine through me in my own unique way.

From below, I heard my mother call, "Bene, it's getting late. Come in and take a shower."

"Yes, Mommy," I answered. However, before I went in, I looked up at the sky and made a promise to myself and to God. I promised that from that day forward, I would cry no more over being different, nor would I let anyone else define me. I would let my light shine through the power that God gives me. I did not yet know what form that might take, but I was still just a boy. I had a long time to figure that out.

Chapter Three

To Be Myself

One cold Sunday afternoon, my family sat down at the dinner table for a Sunday lunch of white rice, steamed spinach, and chicken tomato stew. My brother Chizoba, my sister Mirian—whom we all called Mie-Mie—and I were the only children still living at home. We all loved Sunday lunch because it was the one day of the week we got to drink a bottle of Coca-Cola with our meal. I had just taken my first drink of my Coke when my dad looked over at me and asked with his deep, baritone voice, "Bennet, my son, what do you want to become?"

The answer was easy. "An airline pilot," I said. All my life I had dreamed of becoming a pilot. Sometimes at night, I would lie in my backyard and watch the lights of planes flying across the sky, wondering where they were going. I could see myself at the helm of one of those jumbo jets, flying all over the world. One day I would fly into Paris, where my beautiful Parisian girlfriend waited for me with open arms. The next day might be Sydney, where a gorgeous Australian model awaited me. Of course I would fly across the Pacific to San Francisco where the most beautiful woman in all of America would wrap her arms around me, welcoming me back. I could not imagine a better life.

"A pilot?" my mother yelled out like she'd just discovered a snake under the table. "My son, you will die young in a plane crash. No, you cannot become a pilot!"

Her response surprised me. The beautiful girlfriends in Paris and

Sydney and San Francisco wouldn't do me much good if I were dead. Shaken, I asked, "So what do *you* want me to become?"

My father's baritone voice boomed again. "What about medical school?" This was not a question. In Nigeria in those days, many of the top students went to medical school and became doctors. That was the societal expectation. One of my sisters was already in medical school. One doctor in the family was not enough for my father. He wanted more.

"Yes, sir," I said in my little angelic voice, while inside I was dying. I did not want to become a doctor, but once my father made up his mind about the matter, I had no choice.

I was only fourteen when this conversation took place, but I was close to completing high school. In Nigeria at that time, you could bypass college and go directly to medical school if you passed the entrance exams. I guess I could have purposely failed the entrance exams, but I could not do that to my father. He expected me to try to do my best, and that is what I did. I took the entrance examinations and passed with flying colors. As a result, I got my first choice of schools, which was the College of Medicine at the University of Nigeria in Enugu, Nigeria. Given what happened to me later in life, there have been many days where I looked back and thought I should have stuck to my guns and run away to pilot training school. Instead, at the age of sixteen, I packed my bags and moved away from home to begin med school.

Perhaps it was moving away from home at such a young age, or maybe it was the rigors of medical school—or perhaps a little of both— but I soon found myself battling debilitating depression. The loneliness and isolation I experienced growing up did not suddenly go away when I moved to Enugu to start my training as a physician. If anything, they became worse when I arrived on campus. I was one of the youngest in my class. In truth, I was just a child ill equipped for the strictly regimented and structured life of a medical student, no matter how intelligent I may have been. I did not have the energy or the drive of my peers because I did not want to be there. I did not want to be a doctor. Nothing about the life of a physician appealed to me. In truth, I have many days where it still doesn't. If it had been up to me, the story of my life would have been written in the skies. But the choice of medicine was not up to me. I was there because medical school was where my family wanted me to be.

Given my lack of enthusiasm, it might have been natural for me to shut down and not try. But I could not do that to my father and mother. My only motivation to succeed came from my deep-seated desire not to let them down. In the super-high stress and ultra-competitive world of medicine, that motivation does not last long. Looking back, I cannot help but believe that God chose this path for me, even though it was the last choice I would have made for myself.

Throughout my first year of med school, I managed to keep my grades up and do what was expected of me. I might not have been excited about medicine, but I greatly enjoyed studying science. It fed my natural curiosity and awakened more questions inside of me. All of my life, I had been immersed in faith in God and His Son, Jesus. As I plunged into my medical studies, I did not find science and faith at odds with one another. The more knowledgeable I became in science, the more I realized what I did not know, which still pushes me deeper into my faith in God. The quest of science was and is a quest for truth. The same is true of my faith. All truth is from God, for God is truth. That means science and faith share a common end point, a common outcome, for they both seek truth. For me, faith and science synergize one another. My faith has enhanced my science, and my science has enhanced my faith.

If medical school had allowed me to pursue this passion with none of the other trappings, I might have found joy there. However, I found very little time for quiet contemplation or for allowing my imagination to take flight with the new truths I had learned. Someone once compared the first two years of medical school to trying to get a drink out of a fire hose. If anything, that is an understatement. Information flew at me so fast that I only had time to grab as much as I could as fast as I could and keep moving. This was not a time for self-discovery; it was a time for digesting more information than any human mind could take in, and to do so as quickly as possible.

During my second year of medical school, I began to lose the little energy and drive I had. Every day felt like the day before. I lost interest in my studies and in life. Many days, I could hardly push myself out of bed. I struggled to keep up with my school schedule, a struggle I slowly began to lose.

One Sunday afternoon, the fight became more than I could bear. I had a test the next day, one for which I was not ready. I left my room and started across campus to the library to study my biochemistry textbook. The book was the only thing I had to study. By this point, I had stopped taking notes in class lectures—that is, when I bothered to go to class at all. As I walked across the campus of the University of Nigeria, I noticed all the other students around me, talking and laughing and acting like they didn't have a care in the world. A huge weight seemed to come down upon me. I stopped along the sidewalk and sat down upon a large rock. Just keeping my body upright took all of the energy within me. More people moved around me. All of them, every single one, appeared to have a better life than me. They all seemed to have a reason for living. I didn't.

Once I finally mustered up enough energy to stand up, I stumbled back to my room and collapsed on my bed and did not move for the rest of the day. I failed the exam. My grades in other classes started to plummet. Most days, I could not force myself to get out of bed, much less go to class. Eventually I left school and went to my sister Winny's house in Lagos, about 350 miles west of Enugu. When she asked why I was there, I told her I was on a school break. About the time she became suspicious that mine might not be an official school break, I left and went to a close family friend's house in Jos, which was another 350 miles north of Enugu. I did not socialize with him or his family while there. Most of the time, I stayed in his guest room, in bed, lying in darkness and silence.

I did not yet understand that I was suffering from textbook clinical depression. Today, people ask me why I pushed so hard to find answers for Mike Webster, the Pittsburgh Steelers legend, when he died in 2002. This is the answer. Before I went into work the morning of Mike Webster's autopsy, I watched the news reports about his death. The reporters spoke of how Iron Mike had isolated himself from everyone who had known and loved him. He suffered, they said, from depression and other ailments. I could relate to Mike. More than that, I listened to the tone with which the reporters spoke. They talked down about Mike, as if he had chosen to suffer from depression and the terrors that drove him to my autopsy table at only fifty years of age. Their words made me angry. This man was a child of God—made in God's image, beloved of God. He deserved better. Watching the reports, I saw myself as a young medical student in Mike Webster. Only those who have suffered depression can understand the darkness that descends upon one's soul. That's one of the reasons I believe my meeting him was truly an act of God. The Lord Himself brought the two of us together, two very different men and yet connected by our battles with the darkness of depression.

• • • •

In the middle of my struggle with depression, I tried to reason with myself in an attempt to figure out this dark disease. The more I reasoned and rationalized, the darker my world became. I could not understand the question of why I felt like I did and why this was happening to me. But the more I asked "why me?" the more I realized asking this question was not going to help me overcome the darkness. Instead, I began desperately praying, *God, please help me.* He did not come down to me as an angel to touch my head and heal me, but God did help me. For one thing, I slowly realized that this was going to be a long journey and that I had to be patient with myself. I also reset my expectations of myself. Before this, I expected to achieve top marks in all of my classes. The depression and resulting lack of energy and focus made this next to impossible. That's when I decided that it did not matter if I scored an A or a C, as long as I finished the course and graduated.

I seriously considered dropping out of med school, but I dismissed this thought because I knew it would devastate my parents. Instead, I made up my mind that once I finished and graduated, I would reevaluate my life and decide on the course of action I wanted to take. If I still wanted to become a pilot, then I would pursue it. Or maybe I would go to law school and practice medical law. *Or*, I thought, *perhaps I will become a doctor and use medicine as an avenue to fulfill my lifelong desire to travel to the United States or other developed countries.* Magazines and movies showed life in the West to be very different from life in Nigeria. As a doctor, that world might be open to me. After all, a physician is a physician all over the world. If I could pass the licensing exams from other countries, my medical degree could be my ticket to travel wherever I wanted to go.

Even with my newfound resolution, I had a long, difficult climb to reach my goal. The depression did not leave me simply because I had prayed and asked God for help. My energy levels remained very low. Getting out of bed was a constant battle. When I did make it to class, I could not focus.

The more I struggled, the harder I prayed. One of God's answers to my prayers came in the form of a friend and classmate named Kenneth. A very quiet, soft-spoken Christian guy, Kenneth saw beyond my struggles to see the potential within me. We shared most of the same classes. When I could not make it to class, Kenneth left his lecture notes for me to study. Late at night, as my classmates slept, I stayed up studying the notes, chewing on kola nuts and smoking Șt Moritz cigarettes to stay awake. In the morning I returned his notes to him. Then, when it came time to take my examinations, I passed. Most of my classmates couldn't understand how I could digest all the information without attending class. Only Kenneth and I knew our secret.

However, I faced another hurdle. Several of my classes required that I actually attend to get credit. Without attending the lectures, I could not take the examinations. Kenneth bailed me out there as well. On the days I could not lift the weight of my depression in order to function, he secretly signed my name on the attendance book. I never asked him to do this for me. Why he did it, I will never know. He was simply the angel I needed in my life at that time. I could never have completed medical school without him. Unfortunately, the two of us have lost contact over the years. I hope he knows how great a debt of gratitude I owe to him.

Not all of my classes could be handled in this way, however. One professor in particular required that I make rounds with him to be allowed to pass the class. I tried, but I could not do it. He, in turn, barred me from taking the final examination. Another professor was made aware of my struggles through my sister, Uche, who was already a physician. The professor empathized with me, which was rare in those days. Back then, mental illness carried a stigma and was misunderstood. Through my sister, he let me know that if I attended rounds with him whenever I could, he would make sure I was eligible to take all my exams. Good to his word, I was allowed into the examination of the professor who had previously told me to not bother showing up.

I arrived for my examination right on time. I dove into the test, which was timed, and lost myself in it. Thirty minutes after the testing started, the proctor administering the exam came to me and said, "You must leave the examination room." He then took my examination papers from me.

Shocked, I immediately ran to the second professor and explained the situation to him. He went back to the examination room with me and requested that I be allowed to finish the test. The proctor agreed. Unfortunately, the time I lost while all this took place was lost. I still had to finish the exam at the same time as everyone else. I looked up at the clock. I only had forty-five minutes remaining. *O Lord, help me*, I prayed. I then began answering the multiple-choice questions as quickly as I could. With no time to sit back and think deeply about each question, I circled the first answer that came into my head. In desperate times you do what you have to do.

I passed the test. When I received my grades, I thanked God for the angel He had sent to help me. Without the kindness of the other professor, I would have failed the class and not graduated from medical school.

• • • •

In my final year of medical school, all graduating students were asked to write a short section for the class yearbook. "What are you going to do after medical school?" we were asked. I guess they wanted to have us write out all the great things we hoped to do and accomplish in the future. Some people wrote about how they wanted to become the best neurosurgeon in the whole country. Others spoke of building hospitals in underserved areas of the nation. Still others spoke of moving into administrative positions or curing diseases.

I gave the shortest answer of all my classmates. In answering the question, I wrote just three words: to be myself. I was still trying to figure out who I was as I fought through the fog of depression that had descended upon me, yet I held out the hope that I could find myself there. This was my one desire. I had only this one life as a gift from God. I now had to discover who He had created me to be and then pursue this man with all I had within me. Only then could my light shine for Him.

My answer did not win me any accolades. My classmates looked at me like something was wrong with me. I did not care. I had one desire, and I planned to pursue it. I was going to be myself, no matter who that turned out to be.

Chapter Four

Answered Prayer

When I was ten years old, my father returned to work in Jos, the city where my family lived prior to the Nigerian civil war. My mother, brother, sister, and I stayed behind in Enugu. I couldn't understand what was happening. My father returned home from time to time, and we occasionally visited him in Jos. The first trip there made me angry. In Enugu, we lived in a small rental house in a middle-class neighborhood, or at least middle class for an Igbo family in Nigeria. Such a neighborhood would never be thought of as middle class outside of Nigeria. But my father—he lived in a palace in Jos. The government provided the house to him as part of his job as deputy director of mines. The British built the house many years earlier for colonial administrators from England. Even though the British were gone and Nigeria was an independent nation, the house still carried the perks that the English administrators enjoyed, including a butler, a chef, domestic helps, and even a chauffeur. We stayed with my father during our two-month summer vacation from school, but then it was back to the small rented house in Enugu. To my young mind, this just seemed wrong.

At the time, I had no way of understanding the level of fear my father felt just being in Jos after witnessing the widespread violence against the Igbo in the streets during the civil war. Even ten years later, he could feel the tension that remained between the victorious Hausa people and the losers, the Igbo. He did not encounter as much prejudice, in part because he spoke the Hausa dialect fluently without an accent. Even so, he remained petrified by his experiences during the war. He lost many friends and witnessed the slaughter of his fellow Igbo by the Hausa. No wonder he did not want his family to move permanently to Jos. He had us stay in Enugu for our own safety. The war may have been over, but the deep scars remained.

My young mind could not yet comprehend any of this, although I recognized something was broken in the culture around me. A state of progressive decay had set in, but no one seemed to mind. Mediocrity was the order of the day. School classrooms were filled with litter and remained year after year in a state of disrepair. Yet at the back of the room sat the civil servant whose job it was to keep the place clean. No one seemed to mind that he didn't do his job. Nor did anyone else seem to notice all the days when the water wasn't working and toilets wouldn't flush. Garbage littered the unpaved streets that were filled with ruts and potholes, and yet no one complained. Everyone simply chose to keep quiet and look the other way.

• • • •

Ten years later, when I graduated from medical school, nothing had changed. Nigeria remained in a state of decay, and no one seemed to care. My frustration grew when I entered the mandatory National Youth Service Corps, a Nigerian national program where university graduates engage in service to the country for a year. Because I was now a doctor, I was assigned to work as an emergency room physician in the city of Jos. I also worked part-time as a general practitioner in a family practice clinic. The experience only confirmed my original reluctance to become a doctor. I was not comfortable working with living patients. No matter how many patients I treated and no matter how positively they responded to me, the old feelings of inadequacy always came rushing back to the surface. I really just wanted to fade into the background and be left alone.

More than the discomfort I felt working with patients, my soul was weighed down by the brokenness I saw in the country around me. Every day, I encountered distraught families who carried in their sick children. Many of the children suffered from preventable ailments like malnutrition. *How can we not have enough food for our weakest members?* I wondered. It was as though no one felt it their responsibility to watch out for the society as a whole. As Cain said in Genesis 4:9 when confronted with taking his brother's life, no one felt compelled to be their "brother's keeper." In addition to malnutrition, the children usually came in with malaria or gastroenteritis, vomiting, and passing loose stools. I treated them the best I could, but my efforts failed because more often than not, the hospital did not have the medications my patients needed. As a result, children died needlessly and preventably. But just like with the broken streets and schoolrooms, no one seemed troubled by the system. I could not understand that. I still cannot.

I raised objections to my superiors. At best, other doctors just shrugged their shoulders and said something like, "That's just how things are."

"But that doesn't mean that's how they have to be!" I objected. I know I was young and idealistic, but even now, more than two decades later, I still cannot accept the excuse that "that's just how things are." I encounter this sort of collective ignorance that I call conformational intelligence wherever I go. Frankly, I find it to be one of the greatest barriers to effecting real change in contact sports in America. I find it to be more than simply accepting a bad situation as fait accompli. Rather, conformational intelligence willingly closes one's eyes to the obvious negative outcomes and calls their very existence into question. I could not go along with this when I was a young doctor any more than I can today. I find it maddening.

I define conformational intelligence as a phenomenon whereby the way you think and perceive the world, including your sense of right and wrong and good and evil, are controlled, constrained, and constricted by the expectations, cultures, traditions, norms, and mores of the society around you without you even knowing it or being aware of it. As a result, when objective, factual evidence is presented to you that runs counter to the conformational cast of your mind, you deny and reject that evidence, even though it is true and your preconceived ideas are false.

Some people have told me that if I had grown up in this country and become consumed by the conformational intelligence surrounding football, there was no way I could have performed an autopsy on Mike Webster. I would have been in so much awe of him that I would not have touched his body. Mike Webster had seen some of the best physicians and surgeons in the best hospitals in the United States, but those physicians, because of their conformational fascination, love, and infatuation with football, did not link football with Mike Webster's ailments. It took an outsider like myself, who did not conform to America's cast of the mind about football, to objectively link Mike Webster's ailments to football and identify CTE. Yet when I presented my findings to the same best doctors in the United States, they ridiculed, dismissed, and tried to discredit me and my work because it challenged their cast of the mind about football.

My raising objections to the way things were falling into line with the conformational intelligence around me caused other doctors to see me with suspicious eyes. Yet I could not keep quiet. God and His Spirit within me would not allow me to stay silent. As a child of God and a recipient of life from Him, I owe it to Him to be the best I can be and to glorify Him in all I do. I felt very frustrated that no one else seemed to share this conviction.

The tipping point for me came late one night when a man was rushed into my emergency room. He had just been involved in a car wreck. When he came into the ER, he was awake and alert. However, his vitals started going down quickly. I examined him and discovered he had suffered a major vascular injury in his abdomen and was bleeding internally. However, our hospital did not have a trauma or vascular surgeon available. I called the general surgeon on duty and explained the situation. "If we don't get him into surgery, he's going to die," I said.

"I'll get back to you," the general surgeon said. But he never did. I called back. No answer. For reasons he never felt compelled to explain to me, the general surgeon refused to operate on the young man.

The young man's pain increased as he began to slip in and out of consciousness. I tried to make him comfortable. Apart from performing an operation myself—and I had not been trained in any type of surgery, so doing the operation myself was not an option—there was nothing I could do to help him. Over the next thirty minutes, I stood by the man's bed, helplessly watching his life slip away until death finally took him. His life could easily have been saved, but there was no one in the hospital able to save him.

I knew the system was broken, but I was still young and filled with youthful idealism. I thought the system could be repaired. When Nigeria's leaders scheduled a presidential election for 1993, the first since military dictator General Babangida and others had taken control over the nation in a 1983 coup, I thought real change was just around the corner. The government promised that these would be fair and open elections, true democracy in action. Patterning ourselves after America, two political parties were formed—the Social Democratic Party and the National Republican Convention. I joined the SDP. The SDP candidate for president was a wealthy, charismatic man named Moshood Abiola. He was a billionaire and a member of the Yoruba tribe. Even though he was a Muslim, he was very friendly toward Christians. He grew up in a Christian environment and attended Christian schools. His opponent was a Hausa Muslim, Bashir Tofa, who chose an Igbo man, Sylvester Ugoh, as his vice-presidential candidate.

The election filled our nation with hope. I was so excited by the prospect of a civilian leader who might actually put the people's best interests first that I campaigned for Abiola. This was to be our country's rebirth. International observers were brought in to oversee the election to ensure its fairness. On the day of the election, I went to my assigned polling place. Rather than cast a paper ballot, people lined up in a designated place to show their support for either the SDP or the NRC candidate. Once everyone was in line, representatives from both parties walked down the line, counting the votes. Their results were certified by Western observers. The entire process was carried out in a very orderly fashion. No one rioted. No one cheated. I think we were all too excited by the prospect of actually having our voices heard to even think of trying to silence the other side.

Because of the way the votes were cast, it was obvious on Election Day that Abiola would win easily. Perhaps that was one of the reasons that the election was carried out the way it was. By having each candidate's supporters publicly show their support, no one was going to be surprised by the results. The announced results fell in line with what everyone already knew. I thought that change had finally arrived.

And then, eleven days after the election, the military dictator, General Babangida, suddenly announced in a nationally televised speech that he had annulled the election results. He claimed the election had not been free and fair. Even today, twenty-three years later, Nigerians around the world continue to protest this action. However, at the time, there was nothing we could do. When I heard the announcement, I sat down and wept for my country. I went into my bedroom, shut the door, and cried loudly. Our only hope had been crushed. Instead of a freely elected president, we were stuck with a corrupt government that did not care about its people. I knew right then that there was no future for me in my home country. For me to remain there for the rest of my life would mean conforming to the traditions, norms, mores, and expectations of a corrupt society. It would mean I had accepted the conformational intelligence of that society and fallen into the perspective that this is the way life is going to be. Staying and fighting to change the system was not an option, at least not in the context of my family's and my Igbo people's history. Change had already been attempted, and it ended in disaster.

I felt I had no future in Nigeria, but I believed I knew where my future could be found. As a child, I had discovered a place called the United States of America. America sets you free to be whatever you want to be, to dream and achieve impossible dreams. A place filled with the most intelligent people on earth. I fell in love with America from afar. At night I fell asleep dreaming of the United States, only to awaken each morning in a world where little children died in my care because the hospital where I worked did not have the most basic medicines needed to cure preventable diseases.

• • • •

I wanted to go to America, but I could not just pack my bags and hop on the next plane. The United States makes very few visas available for those who are not immediate relatives of United States citizens. The process of obtaining one of these visas is far more complicated, and far costlier, than I ever could have imagined. (From the time I first entered the United States in 1995 until I became a citizen twenty years later, I spent more than $100,000 on immigration fees, attorney fees, visa application and renewal fees, and related expenses.) I had no idea where to start in the process, so I did what I always do when I need wisdom and guidance: I prayed to God. I did not pray, *God, let me go to America.* Instead I prayed, *Father, let Your Spirit guide me. I do not believe my future lies in Nigeria. You show me where You want me to go. May Your Spirit lead me, and I will follow.*

In addition to prayer, I went to the library and started researching possible places where I could move and pursue my future. I wanted to go to America, but I knew I needed options if it did not work out. Because I was fluent in English, I focused primarily on English-speaking countries. I read books about Australia and New Zealand, both of which appealed to me. New Zealand had a program for doctors to come in and serve underserved minorities in rural areas. Australia had a similar program. I wrote to both countries' embassies and requested application papers. At the same time, I continued exploring ways to get to America.

Unfortunately, my efforts to get to the United States led me nowhere. There wasn't a program to which I could apply. However, to keep my options open, I began studying for the United States Medical Licensing Examination (USMLE). I knew that for me to go to America, God was going to have to throw open the door. However, I also knew that I had to be ready when that door opened. I didn't even need a door. If God just cracked a window of opportunity, I was determined to do the rest. And guess what? He did!

I continued working as an emergency room physician at the university hospital in Jos. My colleagues laughed at me when they saw me studying for the USMLE. "Bennet, you are such a dreamer. You are a single African man. No one is ever going to let you into America. Instead of wasting your time studying for something that is never going to happen, you need to apply to one of the residency programs here in Nigeria," they said to me. Several well-meaning senior physicians pulled me aside and urged me to stop chasing an impossible dream. "You will only come away disappointed and hurt," they said.

Rather than listen to them, I trusted God. I believed that God knew me better than I knew myself. He created me. He knows the number of strands of hair on my head. Before He ever created me, He knew the purpose and plan He has for my life. I believe He placed the aspirations in my heart so that He could place me where He wanted me to go and serve humanity. I had long ago given up my silly childhood dreams of grandeur. I simply wanted to go and do what God had in mind for me. I trusted Him and surrendered my all to Him.

One day, I went into work at the hospital for my afternoon shift. Most days, I was on duty from 2:00 p.m. to 10:00 p.m. and spent all of my time with patients. On this day, I arrived at the hospital early and went through the department, talking with the staff and nurses before going to my office. When I got to my desk, I noticed a letter lying there that did not look like a typical letter. The letterhead and quality of the paper made it clear it had come from an outside country. I grabbed the letter and quickly read it. It came from the World Health Organization in Lyons, France. The letter announced that the International Agency for Research on Cancer had started a fellowship program at several universities in the United States. The IARC pledged to sponsor any candidate who applied and was accepted as a visiting scholar to study the epidemiology of cancer.

After reading the letter, I sank down in my chair in awe. I shared this desk with other busy ER physicians. Our emergency room was a crazy place, with people running in and out constantly. Yet it seemed that this letter had been placed on this desk, undisturbed, just waiting for me to find it. No other physician had grabbed it. It had not fallen on the floor, like most papers on the desks in this room did. I believed that the hand of God placed it right here for me to find.

Because the letter and the program were open to any physician who cared to apply, I made a copy for myself and placed the original on the bulletin board, where all the other doctors could see it. The next day, the letter was gone. I never knew what happened to it.

Over the next two weeks, I went through all the instructions in the letter and did everything the program required. I wrote a letter of intent and attached a copy of my curriculum vitae, and I sent both to the address provided in Lyons. I also sent a copy to the University of Washington in Seattle, which was one of the participating universities. A few months later, I went to my desk at the hospital and found an envelope waiting for me. I picked it up and saw the seal of the University of Washington. I said a quick prayer and opened the letter. "Dear Dr. Omalu," it read, "we are happy to inform you that you have been accepted into the visiting scholar program . . ." I wanted to shout out with joy, but I did not because I was at work. This was nothing less than God at work. He had opened the window. I was going to America. A couple of weeks after I received the letter from the University of Washington, the IARC wrote to inform me that I had received the scholarship which covered the cost of my studies.

God had answered my prayers, but I had no clue as to where I was going. I had no idea where Seattle even was. I even thought it was pronounced "See-tul." All I knew was that it was somewhere in America. My mind had no comprehension of the size and scope of the United States.

Even with the invitation to join the program, I still had more prayers that needed to be answered. The university informed me that before I could start the program, I had to deposit $10,000 in a U.S. bank account, which would cover all my living expenses for the year of study. I may have been a doctor, but I did not make much money. Nor did anyone in my family have an extra ten grand lying around to give me. I went back to prayer. God answered it through my family as a whole. My brother-in-law Sam, my sister Uche's husband, gave me $6,000. My sister Winny's husband, Chuma, gave me $1,000, as did my uncle Remy. I saved up the other $2,000 from my job.

Once I had my money in hand, I thought I was ready to go to America, but my father stepped in and stopped me. "Bennet is too young and immature to go to America and live on his own in a foreign country," he informed my entire family. "He needs to wait one year before he accepts this position." Even though I was twenty-five years old and anxious to get on with life, I realized God was speaking through my father. The University of Washington and the IARC allowed me to defer my entry into the program for one year. The year did not go to waste. I continued studying for, and passed, my USMLE. Now all I had to do was apply for my visa. I assumed the process would be quick and easy. I was about to receive a huge dose of reality. Thankfully, I was also about to learn a lesson about the faithfulness of God and how He turns ordinary people into angels.

Chapter Five

"Heaven Is Here,
and America Is Here"*

Wmultilinehen I told my friends and coworkers I was going to America, they laughed at me. "Don't waste your time," they told me. "The United States will not grant you a visa. I don't know why you are even trying."

"That can't be true," I replied. I had already been invited to come to the United States by the University of Washington and had deposited into a bank all the money I was going to need during my one-year visiting scholar program. *How could I not receive a visa?* I wondered.

"It is true," came the same reply in multiple conversations. Over and over, friends told me, "If you even get an interview in the U.S. Embassy, they won't look you in the eye because you are a single, young, black *Nigerian* man." Apparently, Nigerians had a bad rap internationally, and I did not know it. "The U.S. Embassy officials will just take one look at your passport, stamp it 'rejected,' and tell you to get out. They treat us like animals, not people."

I refused to believe this could be true. However, I still had to recognize what I had heard and act accordingly. I started praying these words from Isaiah 43:

---

*Bennet Omalu made this statement in real life, and it was said by Will Smith, who played Dr. Omalu in the movie *Concussion*.

Remember not the events of the past,

the things of long ago consider not;

See, I am doing something new!

Now it springs forth, do you not perceive it?

In the wilderness I make a way,

in the wasteland, rivers.

Wild beasts honor me,

jackals and ostriches,

For I put water in the wilderness

and rivers in the wasteland

for my chosen people to drink,

The people whom I formed for myself,

that they might recount my praise.[1]

You make a way in the wilderness and rivers in the desert, I prayed. *I know You will make a way for me.*

The time for my visa interview was at hand, which meant I had to travel to Nigeria's most populous city, Lagos, which is where the United States Embassy was located. My sister Winny and her husband lived in Lagos, so I stayed with them while I was there.

The day before my interview, I spent an extended period of time in prayer and reading my Bible. If what I had been told was true, then I needed divine intervention to have any chance of receiving a visa. As I prayed, I felt moved by the Spirit to visit the United States Information Service (USIS) office. The USIS was the American agency that oversaw the exchange visitor program under which fell my visiting scholar program. I did not know if they had anything to do with the visa process, but I felt they should be aware of me and why I was trying to go to America. I did not know if they could help me, but I figured going there could not hurt.

I dressed in my nicest suit, left my sister Winny's house, and took a cab to the USIS office on Lagos Island. When I walked in, I said hello to the receptionist, a young Nigerian woman, and then announced, "I would like to see the director." Why I chose the director rather than any of the other staff members there, I cannot say. The Spirit that lives within us is a bold Spirit, and I believe He directed me.

The receptionist gave me a perplexed look and asked, "Do you have an appointment?"

"No, I do not," I replied.

Skeptical, she asked, "Why do you need to see the director?"

I pulled my file out of my bag. "I am a doctor in Jos. I have been granted a scholarship by the International Agency for Research on Cancer in Lyons, France, to go to the University of Washington in Seattle as a visiting scholar for one year. I hope to apply to a PhD program after that. I have an appointment at the U.S. Embassy tomorrow for a visa interview."

The receptionist gave me a look that said *"you* are a doctor?" Back then I had a baby face and looked much younger than my years. "Hold on just a minute," she said. She picked up her phone and made a quick call. When she hung up, she said, "Go down that hall. The director's secretary will see you."

I walked down to the director's office, where I was greeted by a man and a woman, both in their thirties and both Nigerians. When I introduced myself, the man recognized my name. He attended the same church as my brother Ikem. "Is the director expecting you?" he asked.

"No," I replied. I took out my papers and explained my situation. Both were extremely sympathetic. The woman looked through her appointment book. "The director should be in soon, and he has an open- ing in his schedule. If you can wait, I can arrange for you to see him."

"Thank you. Yes, I will wait," I said. The man told me the director was new, which worked in my favor. Being new on the job, he had not yet had any negative experiences in the country to prejudice his view of Nigerians.

I took a seat on one of the sofas in the office and waited. And waited. And waited. As I waited, I prayed, *Jesus, I love You. All I have is Thine. Yours I am, and Yours I want to be. Do with me what Thou wilt.*

An hour later, a very friendly, slightly overweight man walked into the room. Sticking out his hand to shake mine, he introduced himself as the USIS director and said, "Come into my office and have a seat."

I followed him into his office and handed him my file. When I explained my situation, he seemed surprised to hear that I was a doctor. I went through the entire process I had followed to land both the scholarship and my entry into the visiting scholar program. As I talked about the visa process and my upcoming interview, he looked through my papers, listening intently, not saying a word. When I finished, he looked up at me, rather puzzled, and said, "How can I help? I'm not really involved in the visa process."

I looked him in the eye and said, "I have been told that my visa application will probably be denied because I am a young, black Nigerian male. That is not right. I have diligently followed all the instructions given me. I have fulfilled all criteria required of me. All of my documents are together. Nothing is lacking. I therefore see no reason why I should be denied an entry visa. I want to go to America not to take, but to give. I have much to offer in service to the country."

"I agree," the director said. He looked over my papers for a few more moments. "I tell you what," he said. "Go to your visa interview tomorrow, and I fully believe you will receive your visa without a problem. However, if you are denied, come back and see me."

"Okay, thank you," I said. Not wanting to take any chances, I then asked, "Would you call the embassy and explain my situation to them?"

"No, that won't be necessary," he said. "I need not interfere in the process. But if you are denied, you come back and see me."

"Thank you so much," I said and left.

• • • •

The next morning, I woke up very early. I did not have time for prayer. I had to be at the United States Embassy by 5:00 a.m. Why they chose such an early hour, I do not know. The American Embassy did not exactly go out of its way to be accommodating toward Nigerians in those days.

I caught a cab and arrived at the embassy before the sun was up. A long line snaked across the front of the building. I walked over to the line and asked someone next to me what was going on. "Why such a long line?" I asked. "I thought I had an appointment."

"It's like this every day," the person replied. "They make us stand outside like this in the dark or in the hottest part of the day. It doesn't matter. Even when it pours down rain, we have to stand outside, waiting our turn to get in. It is like we are not even human."

"That's not right," I said.

The person just laughed. "Then this must be your first trip to the American Embassy."

I stood in line for an hour. The sun came up, and the temperature quickly rose. Finally someone from the embassy stepped out and said, "Bennet Omalu."

"Right here," I said.

"Follow me," the person said and walked into the building without waiting to see where I was.

Once inside, I found a place to wait in a large lobby. Other people waited as well. Ten or fifteen minutes later, a young American woman called my name and case number through a speaker from behind a thick glass window like you would find in a highly secured bank in a poor, crime-ridden inner-city neighborhood. I walked over to the window and noticed there was no chair or stool for me to sit upon. The young woman behind the glass sat above me and looked down at me. I could not tell if she was black or white. I could only tell she was American. Perhaps I was too nervous to see much else. The thickness of the glass also made it hard to see her clearly.

"Passport," she said without emotion. I passed it through the small slot at the bottom of the window.

"Do you have your documents?" she asked without looking up. I passed them through the slot. She flipped through the papers very quickly, one after another. If she was reading them, she had to be the fastest reader on the planet.

"How long do you hope to stay in the United States?" she asked, again without looking at me.

"One year," I replied.

"You're a doctor?" she asked with a tone that made it clear she did not believe me.

"Yes. I graduated from—"

Before I could finish my answer, she said, "Thank you," in a way that didn't sound like she was thanking me for anything. She then pushed the papers back into a stack, pulled out a rubber stamp from a drawer, and banged it down on the top page of my documents and on a page in my passport. "Visa denied," she said as she signed the paper. She pushed all my papers back through the slot and said, "You may file a petition to have your denial reviewed," in a voice that sounded like an answering machine recording.

"But I have—"

"Thank you, NEXT," she said looking past me as she waved me off.

• • • •

I walked out of the embassy and back onto the streets of Lagos. A long line of people stood in the heat waiting their turn to go in and be denied. I wondered why anyone bothered applying for a visa. Everything anyone had ever told me about the U.S. visa process had been confirmed. Never had I felt so dehumanized. Stopping at a pay phone, I called my family and told them what had happened. "What are you going to do now?" my brother Ikem asked.

"I guess I will go see the USIS director. I don't know what else I can do," I said.

I caught a cab and went straight to the USIS office. When I walked in, the two assistants to the director I had met the day before acted like they were expecting me. "The director told me to come back to see him if my visa was denied," I explained. "It was, so here I am."

Both the assistants nodded knowingly as I spoke, as if they had already been told I was going to be denied. "The director is out right now," the man said, "but you may wait for him." He said it in a way that made me think they had already contacted the director and let him know I needed to see him.

For two hours I sat and waited. Those may have been two of the darkest hours of my life. Everything for which I had worked for so long now appeared to have been yanked out of my hands. I was afraid. *Why did I even try?* I wondered. My coworkers' words echoed in my ears. *How can I go back and face them? They will never let me hear the end of this.* The scene from the embassy replayed in my mind over and over. *How can my fate, my entire future, rest in the hands of one person? It cannot. My fate, my future, rests in the hands of God.* I began to pray aloud, *Jesus, I love You. All I have is Thine. Yours I am, and Yours I want to be. Do with me what Thou wilt.* I started to wonder if God's will might be Australia or New Zealand. *If this falls through, I will try them next. Don't worry. This is not the end.*

My brother Ikem called his friend in the USIS office as I sat there. He just wanted to make sure I was still there and that I had not gone off somewhere to harm myself. My family was genuinely worried about me. I had put all my hope into going to the United States. They did not know what I might do if I were forced to remain in Nigeria and give up my dream forever.

After my two hours of waiting, the USIS director came running into the office. Sweat poured off of him, and he was out of breath. When he saw me, he stopped dead in his tracks. "Bennet, what are you doing here?" he asked.

"They denied my visa," I replied.

"What?" he said, shocked. "Follow me." I walked with him into his office. He sat down next to me and picked up his phone. After a few moments, he said into the phone, "Consular office, please. Yes, I'll hold." When the consul picked up on the other end, the director said, "Hola." He then began speaking in a language I did not recognize. Later—as in years later—I figured out he was speaking Spanish. I guess he did so to keep me from hearing the whole conversation. Apparently the director was Hispanic. Back then, he just looked white to me. In Nigeria, everyone was either white, black, or Asian. I was not nearly as conscious of race then as I am now.

After a five-minute conversation, the director hung up the phone and scribbled a note on a piece of paper. He slipped it into an envelope and handed it to me. On the front of the envelope he wrote the consul's name. "Take this back to the embassy. Show it to the guards at the gate, and they will let you right in. Hurry. They're expecting you, and the office will close soon."

"Thank you so much," I said. I rushed back to the embassy and did exactly what I had been told. Rather than make me wait in line, a guard ushered me right in. I went inside the embassy and walked right past the large lobby ringed with glass-windowed cubicles where everyone else had to do their business. The guard led me to the consular office, where I was invited to wait on a very comfortable sofa. All around me, people came and went. I sat quietly. A half hour later, a lovely African-American woman appeared out of nowhere. "Are you Bennet?" she asked with a smile.

"Yes," I said, a little startled.

"May I have your passport?" she said, not even asking for the rest of my documents. As I handed it to her, she said, "I think you know my daughter." She gave me her daughter's name, which I no longer remember. "She was in medical school with you. She came here from America, but being so far from home was hard for her, so she went back."

The name was very familiar to me then. "Yes, I know her. Such a lovely girl." The two of us then talked about her daughter like we were two old friends. I sympathized with her over her daughter going back to the States. "I nearly quit myself more than once," I said. We talked like this for about five minutes. Finally the woman smiled and said, "If you come back tomorrow afternoon at two, your passport and visa will be ready for you."

"Oh, thank you—thank you so much!" I said. By now it was nearly dark, so I rushed back to my sister's house, so excited and nervous that I could hardly eat or sleep. The next day at two o'clock, I had my passport with the visa stamp in my hand. I called the USIS office to thank the director, but he was not in, so I left a message. The next day I called again but still could not reach him. I should have gone back and thanked him in person, but I never did. He truly was an angel from God for me.

• • • •

I returned to Jos and immediately resigned from my job at the hospital. Suddenly my colleagues who had laughed at me for wanting to go to America now came to me asking for advice. "What should I do to get a visa too?" they asked. I didn't have any advice to give them. God had opened this door for me. He would have to do the same for them.

Even though my visa was only good for a year, I did not plan on returning to Nigeria. Already I had started thinking of applying to the PhD program at the University of Washington. If accepted, my visa could easily be extended. Since I did not plan on returning to Nigeria, I spent my last couple of weeks in the country of my birth giving away all my possessions. I didn't have a lot. Most things went to my family, but I also gave treasured items to friends. Giving my things away made the reality of going to America seem real. I was like the old Spanish explorer Hernán Cortés dismantling my ships before my plane even got off the ground.

I flew back to Lagos before departing for America. I stopped over for one night at my sister Winny's house. That night, I enjoyed my last meal in Nigeria. Right before I left for the airport, my two sisters, Winny and Uche, along with my brother Ikem, gathered in Winny's living room. A couple of years earlier, Winny and Ikem had become evangelical Christians. We worshiped together in their living room, singing songs of praise. They also read Scripture passages over me and laid their hands on me, asking God to cover me with the blood of Jesus as I went out on this new adventure. I will never forget Winny's prayer over me. She prayed, "God, if there is anything that will make Bennet turn away from You, please take that thing away from him. No man or woman created by the mighty God can deny Bennet his blessings. And we claim Bennet's blessings in the MIGHTY NAME OF JESUS!"

My eyes filled with tears as Winny prayed. I felt like heaven had come to earth in that living room. But I could not sit and take it all in. I had to get to the airport. Time was now against me. When I rushed out the front door, I felt the presence of the Holy Spirit. I walked out toward the waiting car with Winny. Ikem was driving. I looked up at the empty blue sky and thought back to how I used to wait for night to fall so that I could see the lights of the jumbo jets streaking across the sky from the international airport. Every light made me wonder where the plane was going. Europe? America? And I always wondered if someday I might be on one of those planes. Now that day had come.

On the way to the airport, we ran into a terrible traffic jam. Lagos has the worst traffic I've seen anywhere in the world. Most days it did not present a problem for me. Today it did. Cars, trucks, and buses were all at a standstill. I glanced down at my watch. "I hope I don't miss my plane," I said.

"What time is it?" Winny asked. I showed her my watch. "This isn't going to work," she said. "Let's go."

"Where?" I asked. "We're already in the car."

"Just follow me," she said. Winny jumped out of the car, opened the trunk, and pulled out my luggage. Looking around, she saw a couple of motorcycle cabs called okadas. She hailed two. The okadas could weave in and out of the traffic and go places when no one else could. "Get on the second bike and follow me," she said. Winny then took my luggage, placed it on top of her head, straddled the first motorcycle, and told the driver, "Get to the airport as fast as you can." I nearly fell off the second motorcycle laughing at the sight of my sister balancing on the okada with my suitcase on her head.

Winny's plan worked. In less than thirty minutes, we arrived at the airport. The two of us didn't have time for a long good-bye. Tears ran down my face. I don't know if they were tears of sadness at leaving my family or tears of joy that I was going to America. Either way, there was no time to think. We hugged, and I ran into the airport and toward my gate. Security lines did not exist back then, which allowed me to get to my gate just in time for my flight's scheduled departure. On the flight sign, I saw the words, "Delayed: two hours." That gave me time to go back and say a proper good-bye to my sister and brother. My brother Ikem arrived just as I did. We hugged and cried, and then I said good-bye. Walking away, I turned and waved to them. As hard as it was to leave them, I could not wait to get on with my journey. I could hardly wait to discover what awaited me in America.

I went to the departure lounge inside the airport, got a drink, and sat down to calm my nerves. I raised my glass and gave a toast to God. "Thank You," I said. I felt relieved that God had answered so many prayers for me, but from this point forward, He wouldn't need to help me so much. I was on my way to God's own country—America, the heavenly country. God could now go help some other lost child. I was going to be fine in the place to which He had already given so much.

Chapter Six

Welcome to America

When I boarded the Swissair jumbo jet in Lagos on October 23, 1994, I believed all my troubles were behind me. The flight first landed in Geneva, Switzerland, and then flew eleven hours to Los Angeles International Airport. Once I was on the ground, it did not take long for me to realize I may have left all my troubles in Nigeria, but a whole new set awaited me in America. I spoke English, and I thought my father had well prepared me for the cultural changes I was to encounter here. After all, he had spent four years in England while attending college. He spoke often about the differences between Nigeria and the English-speaking world.

Unfortunately, my father left out a few crucial details, beginning with what was quickly becoming an urgent problem. After landing in Los Angeles, I needed to use the bathroom before I caught my connecting flight to Seattle. In Nigeria, bathrooms are called toilets. Walking through the airport concourse, I searched for a sign that read "Toilet," to no avail. I only saw signs that read "Bathroom" or "Restroom." Since I did not need to take a bath and I did not need to rest, I kept walking. I needed a toilet, and the longer it took to find one, the greater the sense of urgency became. I walked up to a white couple. "Excuse me, can you direct me to a toilet?" I asked. They kept walking and acted like they did not hear me. I approached another white man who was standing over to one side. "Sir, can you help me find the toilet?" He looked at me like I was from Mars.

I approached a handful of other people. All sidestepped me or ignored me or gave me a look that said, "Go away." No one helped me. I did a quick check of my breath to see if it so offended people that I drove them away. All the while, the need to urinate had reached crisis proportions. I stood in the middle of the concourse, unsure what to do next. I danced a bit and grabbed at my crotch like a three-year-old boy who waits until the last possible moment to put down his toys and relieve himself.

Finally, an older Hispanic woman who worked for the airport as a housekeeper came over to me. She had a garbage bag in her hand. "Sir, do you need to find a place to pee?" she asked.

"Yes. Desperately," I said.

"Follow me," she said. Thankfully she walked fast. She led me to a sign marked "Men's Restroom." "Go inside, and you will find a toilet," she said.

The sign did not make sense, but I did not have time to think very deeply about it. I dashed inside, looked around, and found what I was looking for just in time. *Okay*, I said to myself, *restroom means toilet. I must remember that.* I had just learned my first cultural lesson in America.

After relieving myself, I went out and found the woman who had directed me to the restroom. "Thank you!" I said.

"You are welcome," she said with an accent. I did not ask her about her situation, but her accent told me that she had come to the United States from another country and could therefore relate to my cultural confusion.

I had another quick "you're not in Nigeria anymore" moment before I got on my plane bound for Seattle. As I walked to my gate, I saw two people in a passionate embrace, who then engaged in a very long kiss. I didn't say anything, nor did I stare. Their business was their business, not mine. However, I did think to myself, *That's something you never see in Nigeria.* In my home country, people reserve such shows of affection for the privacy of their own home. I got another shock as I glanced back at the couple. It was not a man and woman kissing, but two men. A little voice in my heart said, "Bennet, welcome to America."

• • • •

My flight to the Seattle-Tacoma International Airport landed around 9:30 at night. I walked off the plane with $250 in my pocket. The secretary of the Department of Epidemiology at the University of Washington was waiting at the gate for me, along with another African postgraduate student. I think he was from Zaire or the Congo or the Central African Republic. I don't remember which. They took me to the house where the other grad student stayed. He introduced me to the owners of the house, an elderly white woman and her blind, middle-aged son. They had an attic room they said I could rent for about $30 for the night. Not knowing where else to go, I took it. Later I rented the room for about $180 a month.

My new temporary home sat in a predominantly white neighborhood not far from the university. The location was perfect, although the room was cramped and the bed quite small, even for a small man like me. Nevertheless, I took it. Before I left Nigeria, my father and mother had advised me not to judge things on face value. Things that glitter and look wonderful to the eye may not be good for me; therefore I must be careful. This room definitely did not glitter, but it was everything I needed. That's why I took it.

Classes started right after I arrived in Washington. Very quickly I found myself caught up in the frantic pace of classes, seminars, and assignments. I worked to keep up, while also adapting to a very different culture from the one in which I had spent my entire life. Even in the midst of the hustle and bustle of the university, I felt very lonely. The depression that I had wrestled with for so long returned. That surprised me. I believed that once I came to America, with the hope of a new life, my depression would leave and never return. Perhaps I needed to rethink the idea of leaving God's help behind in Nigeria.

Not every surprise in my new home was negative. There was a grocery store near my house I went to daily because I did not have a refrigerator. My jaw dropped the first time I walked in the store. Never before had I seen such variety and quality. One entire wall had nothing but bread on it. White bread. Wheat bread. Sourdough bread. Low-fat bread. Non-fat bread. Bread, bread, and more bread. What an amazing place to live!

I soon discovered a dark side to this amazing place. My first few times in the store, I was so overwhelmed trying to navigate my way around that I did not notice one of the store employees following me. I only noticed him when he asked if I needed any help. "No, thank you," I said and went on my way.

The next time I was in the store, the same employee followed me around. Once again he asked if I needed any help. I gave the same answer. I noticed he continued following me anyway. Again, he asked if I needed help. I noticed he asked with a false smile on his face—the kind that people put on to appear sincere when they are anything but.

After a couple of weeks of the same employee following me around the store, I began to suspect something was up. I looked around, and it finally hit me: I was the only person of color in the store, and the only one being followed. I also noticed a difference in the way the cashier spoke to me when I paid for my groceries. Those in line in front of me were greeted with a warm smile and a sunny "hello." When it was my turn, I received a suspicious look and a grunt.

The people in the predominantly white neighborhood also acted strangely around me. Several times I noticed people crossing over to the other side of the street when I approached them on the sidewalks. When I walked down the street at night, cars switched on their high beams.

Police cruisers sometimes followed me very slowly down my street. Often the officer pulled up to me and started asking questions like, "Where are you going? What is your business in this neighborhood?" I answered all the questions as politely as I could. I assumed they asked everyone they did not recognize the same sort of questions. However, even after it should have been clear I was no stranger in this neighborhood, the questions from police officers did not stop. Several times I had the same policeman pull up next to me, stop me, and fire away the exact questions he had asked the night before. *Surely he knows by now I belong here*, I thought, but I never said it. Something about the tone of the officers' voices told me not to object too strongly.

The university should have been the one place where I was treated like everyone else, but it was not. Professors routinely ignored me in class when I tried to answer questions. On the rare occasions when they did recognize me, they often put down my answers with a very condescending tone. Other students made comments about me as I passed them in the hall or in the library. The first couple of times it happened, I passed it off as no big deal. When it kept happening, I decided something bigger was at play. It wasn't just the white students who did this. African-American students also seemed to shun me. They would not talk to me or associate with me. I could not figure out why. This did not stop in Seattle. Several years later, during my fellowship in Pittsburgh, one day I walked into the office and discovered a note on my desk that read, "Why don't you go back to the jungle where you belong." This was not the America I had imagined.

After I had been in Seattle for several weeks, I went to the elderly woman from whom I rented the room. I often went to her for answers, like the time I purchased an item at the store for $2.99 but I had to pay more than three dollars. "Why did the store overcharge me?" I asked. She laughed and explained sales tax to me. This time I went to her and explained all I had experienced with the people at the local store, along with the way the police followed me and how people avoided me on the street. "Have I done something wrong?" I asked. "There must be some explanation for what has happened."

The woman asked, "The people who crossed the street when they saw you coming—they were white, right?"

"Yes," I said, unsure of what she was implying. "Why would that matter?"

She laughed a very loud laugh. "Oh, Bennet, welcome to your America."

I had no idea what she was trying to say. "What are you talking about?" I asked.

Rather than explain herself, she told me to go to the university library the next day and check out some history books that covered the American Civil War, as well as the civil rights movement. "Start with the Civil War," she said.

"There was a civil war *here*?" I asked. This was the first I had ever heard of such a thing.

She laughed again. "Your understanding of America is so naively pure," she said. "Yes, there was a civil war fought in the late nineteenth century, in large part over the question of slavery."

Now I thought she had to be messing with me. "What are you talking about? Slavery? How could there be slavery in America, a country founded on freedom?"

"Read the books" was all she said in reply.

The next morning, I got up early and headed over to the university library. I checked out the books she'd recommended and devoured them quickly. I had no idea what to expect when I started reading. What I discovered that day and over the course of the next several days of reading was, to say the least, very disappointing, if not outright offensive. At first I became angry. Very angry. Then I felt betrayed. Finally, I just felt very, very disappointed. The place I thought God had blessed more than any nation on earth—the place where I believed people were intelligent and had learned to overcome the hatred and prejudice that had nearly destroyed my people back in Nigeria, this country I had put just one notch below heaven—was no different from any other place on earth. I had never heard of the practice of chattel slavery, where people were treated like animals, until I read about it in an American history book. Even the slavery of history, like that the Israelites suffered prior to the exodus, allowed slaves to maintain some shred of human dignity. Nor had I ever heard of racism until I experienced it firsthand and then read about its root causes.

By the time I finished reading that day, I was depressed. Not only was my image of America shattered, but my faith in the human race was shaken. *If this is the real America, what hope is there? If people with such freedom, people who have been so blessed by God, have such a dark side, can any place be made perfect?* In part, I had left Nigeria because I was so disappointed by the blind acceptance of injustices and how everyone seemed to go along with conditions and problems that no thinking person should ever accept. Now I found the same attitude in America concerning race.

But there was more to my frustration and anger and depression than simply losing faith in America. I now realized that many people I encountered from this point forward—casually, personally, and professionally—would prejudge me based on the color of my skin and the accent with which I speak. I was going to be marginalized for being a black man and for being an African immigrant. Moreover, I was expected to conform to the expectations of this society where I had to live my life at the mercy of another person's conscience. If a police officer asked me thirty times what I was doing in a neighborhood, I had to smile and take it and answer politely. It was like living in postwar Nigeria all over again, reminiscent of how Igbos were treated like losers. Here the message was, "You are less because of the color of your skin—and you are much less because you are not an American." I had refused to accept this attitude as a child. I had moved to America to get away from it. And now it was here, just as strong and just as evil.

Human beings frequently choose to deny or distort the truth for personal aggrandizement and financial gain, to attain some personal or group objective to the detriment of that common humanity we all share. And in so doing, they use other human beings as pawns. They attempt to define and diminish other people, telling them who and what they should be, where they can go, and how high they can climb. Such a way of life would no doubt rob me of who I am. I refused to become a victim of it and chose to stand firmly rooted in the symbol of who I am—my faith and the truth. Little did I know that this faith would be challenged and confronted by the culture of football and the NFL that was hiding in a nook further down the road of my American journey.

I did not leave the house for a couple days. I didn't go to school. I didn't do anything except sit in my small room on my very small bed and drink to numb the pain and frustration I felt.

When I finally had enough of feeling sorry for myself, the Spirit was able to break through and push me to do here what I had done in my native country. I decided I could not and would not allow myself to be defined by another person. Death would be preferable to such a fate. I made up my mind to never allow another human being created in the image of God to tell me, a child of God, what I could or could not do or where I could or could not go based on the amount of melanin in my skin. Am I not also created in God's image? Is there not one God who created us all? There is not a white God or a black God or an American God or an African God. There is *only one God*, the creator of us all, before whom we all stand equal at His feet.

Nor would I allow anyone to dictate how intelligent I should be or to define and control my life or the opportunities available to me. They could not define my happiness or my joys. I refused that.

My resolution was soon put to the test.

• • • •

I returned to the university and did my best to focus on the program I had entered. Even though this was a one-year program, I had thoughts of entering the PhD program and making epidemiology my primary career focus. One day, I met one of the professors in the program for the first time. "Let me show you around," he said. The two of us went to his research laboratory, where three doctoral students were hard at work. The professor interrupted their work and said, "Guys, I want to introduce you to Bennet Omalu from Nigeria. He thinks he can do what we do." The three students then laughed a very sarcastic laugh.

Anger rose up inside of me, but it went away as quickly as it had come. Instead a thought came to me, a revelation as if a huge curtain had just been lifted from in front of me. *These people are living a lie*, I realized. The revelation came from God Himself. *They are living a lie*, I felt God say to me. *They want you to believe you are inadequate and inferior, and they will do everything they can to feed this lie to you until you believe it yourself. But*

you are My child. My Spirit and My power reside within you. You are not less.
Never let anyone tell you that you are.

This moment was a real turning point for me. Rather than allow myself to be sucked into a lie, I chose to pursue the light of truth. I went back to my father's experience. This son of an orphan—an orphan who suffered abuse and marginalization all his life—was going to take the same path toward truth that my father took. My father went from a three-year-old living on the streets to a college-educated engineer through education, education, and education. All my life he told me, "Education is power, and knowledge is power. When you have knowledge, it is yours, and no one can take it away from you." I left that laboratory and made up my mind to follow my father's example. Education was going to be my path toward overcoming the lies that express themselves through prejudice and racism.

I threw myself into my studies, and not just in my academic field. I read everything I could lay my hands upon to help me understand American society. What I found greatly encouraged me. In fact, I became as excited as I had been downcast a few weeks earlier. I learned that opportunities for education are more abundant and easier to take advantage of here than in most parts of the world. As a fairly new arrival in the United States, I did not have any money, nor did I have social connections. But I discovered that if I was willing to work hard and apply myself, doors would open.

Now the only question I needed to answer was which path I should pursue. I already had a medical degree and had passed the USMLE, which made me eligible to enter an American residency program and pursue a career in medicine. But one of the reasons I entered the visiting scholar program in epidemiology related to cancer was to get away from the clinical side of medicine. I practiced medicine in Nigeria for four years and remained just as uncomfortable working with patients on my last day as I had been on my first. If I applied to the PhD program related to the program I was in at the University of Washington, I would be accepted. As the initial year of study went by, I discovered that this program was not really me.

What, then, to study?

I didn't have a lot of time to make up my mind. My initial visa was due to expire with the conclusion of the one-year visiting scholar program. I had to be accepted into a new program of study before that happened, or I would be on my way back to Nigeria. It took a miracle to get me to America the first time. I didn't want to go back and have to have another miracle to bring me back.

Medicine remained my only real option, which meant I had to start applying to residency programs within the United States right away. Yet that raised another question: In what field should I specialize? I wanted to find a specialty that was as far away as possible from clinical medicine. The only two options I could see in 1994 were radiology and pathology. Radiology would still put me in contact with patients, but to a much lesser degree than other specialties. My research, however, found that very few doctors with medical degrees from outside the United States land radiology residency offers.

That left pathology as the only real path available to me if I were to pursue entering a medical residency program within the United States. To be honest, I was no more enthusiastic about entering a residency program in pathology than I had been in going to medical school at the age of sixteen. The process of elimination is a poor way to choose one's career path. Therefore, I made a bargain with myself. I decided to apply to pathology programs, complete the five years of residency, and apply for fellowship training in whichever field of pathology I found I could best tolerate. After that, I would go on to law school. I could work as an attorney, perhaps focusing on personal injury, wrongful death, or medical malpractice cases. Spending the next five years studying to become a pathologist then looked like the perfect next step to achieving my ultimate goal.

And that's all pathology was ever meant to be—a next step, not a career. Yet, as my father's name always reminded me, you never know what tomorrow may bring. I would soon discover the tomorrow God had in store for me to be filled with surprises.

Chapter Seven

Through the Wilderness

Early on in my faith journey, I had many doubts. Through my teenage years and on into my twenties, doubt was as much a part of my life as faith. It was not my study of science that caused me to doubt God. If anything, the deeper I dove into science, the more I saw the wonders of God. The more I learned, the more I realized I did not know. I plunged myself deeper into the abyss of knowledge, only to discover the waters are deeper than my mind could ever imagine. And to me, the end of the pursuit of knowledge has always brought me to the same destination: God. He is the end of all knowledge. While faith seeks God's truth through the revelation of Himself through His Word and in our souls, science seeks the truth behind the designs and secrets of the physical universe; both pursuits lead to the same destination. All truth is God's truth, and all truth leads back to Him. I never doubted that.

No, the doubt with which I wrestled surrounded one of the essential truths of Christianity: Why did Jesus, the Son of God, the One who is preeminent in all things in heaven and on earth, why did He take on the form of an ordinary man and come to earth to suffer? Why did He allow Himself to be humiliated, dehumanized, and ridiculed? Why did He choose to experience the cross of Calvary, to die such a slow, agonizing, and painful death? From my limited perspective, I thought that since He is God, there had to be other more humane, more reasonable ways for Him to redeem all of mankind without having to experience the cross of Calvary. Why Calvary, and why the cross? Why did saving the human race from our sin demand that the Son of God suffer?

Surprisingly, my doubts began to lift when I started to experience life's hardships, difficulties, and challenges. When I came face-to-face with man's inhumanity to himself and to others, the answers to my doubts about the cross began to come to me. The answers weren't exactly in the form of a why as much as a calling to follow Christ's example. When I encountered racism or bigotry, I went back to the story of the cross. There I saw His arrest, the mock trial, His flogging, and His carrying His cross up Calvary. Then I watched the soldiers put the nails in His hands and His feet. Through it all, He submitted Himself to the will of His Father. By faith and in hope, He totally surrendered to His suffering. As one who professes faith in Jesus, I must now totally surrender in faith, like Jesus, to the pain and darkness and humiliation I face in life. Only then, as I surrender in humility and strength, will I emerge victorious as Jesus did when He rose from the dead. The pain and suffering are not the end of the story. In Jesus' resurrection, we are guaranteed victory. But like everything in life, you never know how strongly you believe something until it is put to the test.

• • • •

After I decided to pursue a residency in pathology to continue my training in the United States, I still had to be matched to a program. To do that, I had to first apply to different medical school residency programs. Before I came to the United States, I had to deposit $10,000 to cover all my expenses for my one year of study. I thought the money would last much longer than a year, but when I began my classes at the University of Washington, I quickly realized I was computer illiterate. I could not even type. This placed me at a huge disadvantage in comparison to the other students. The only way to learn computers is through experience, which led me to take a huge risk. One day, I went to the local computer store and picked out a desktop computer. I also purchased several software packages, including Microsoft Office and a typing program. By the time I walked out of the computer store, I had spent close to $4,000. You must remember that computers were much more expensive in 1995 than they are today. Not many people owned their own personal computers, but I was so desperate to catch up that I was willing to pay any price.

Looking back, I am extremely thankful I made this investment. However, spending 40 percent of all the money I had in the world created a new problem. I needed to do something to make more. On top of that, if I was going to have the money to cover the residency program application expenses and to have the money to travel to wherever I needed to go for the interviews in places where I hoped to match, I had to find a part-time job.

I came across a notice on one of the bulletin boards on campus. "Housekeeper wanted. 10–15 hours per week. $6.00 per hour." I pulled the notice down and called the number on the bottom. No one answered, so I left a message. Apparently there had not been a line of people waiting to land this job. The homeowner called me back and immediately hired me. I had called about other jobs, but this was the first and only one where anyone bothered to call me back.

When I reported for work the first day, I discovered the house was a large Victorian home with five bedrooms. The owner, an older Chinese woman, rented the rooms to students. She took one look at me, gave a sort of disgusted grunt, and said, "Follow me." She took me to where she kept the cleaning supplies. "You can use these, but you better believe I know how much is in here and how much you should use. I keep track." It took me a moment to realize she was implying she thought I might steal some of her supplies. She then led me to the bedrooms I was supposed to clean. As she led me into the first room, she described how she wanted the room cleaned, but she used words and a tone that one might use to someone with no education and no sense. I needed the work, so I just sloughed it off.

I went to work cleaning the rooms she assigned to me that day. When I finished the first, she went in and exploded. "Get back in here!"

she yelled. I did as I was told. "I see a smudge on that window," she said in a very hateful tone. "How can you call a room clean when there is a smudge on the window?" She then proceeded to find fault with everything else I had done in the room. I offered to redo it, but she said, "I'm not paying you to do the same work twice. Leave it. I'll come back and finish it myself."

"Do you want me to keep cleaning the other rooms?" I asked.

"Yes, I want you to keep cleaning. I didn't hire you to stand around and talk, did I?" She then called me something in Chinese that I did not understand, but I had a pretty good idea she wasn't saying, "Good job."

I went back to work. Like everything I strive to do, I did the work as close to perfectly as I could. In spite of her complaints, the woman must have liked the work I did because she called me to come back and clean other rooms the next week. And the next. And the next. However, every time I went to work, she always spoke down to me and cursed at me and found fault with everything I did. But she paid me the $6.00 an hour, just as she promised, and for that I was thankful.

About a month after I started working as a housekeeper, I was at work scrubbing some stains off the floor when a new tenant walked into the house to drop off her bags. Like me, she was an international graduate student. She was from China. When she saw me down on the floor scrubbing away, she gave me a very puzzled look. The homeowner was close by, criticizing my work as usual. The student paused for a moment and then asked, "Aren't you a student at school?"

I gave a very muffled "yes, how are you?"

The student then turned to the homeowner and said, "He's a graduate student in the school of public health with me."

The homeowner's eyes got wide, as if the girl's words had collided with all she had assumed about me and was now about to make her head explode.

The student turned back to me. "I know a little about you. You are a doctor, right?"

"Yes, I am," I said very quietly.

That did it. My boss looked at me like she'd just seen a ghost. The look was a mixture of shock, surprise, and embarrassment over the way she had treated me.

I finished my work, received my pay for the day, and never went back. I was very embarrassed for the woman. She called me the next day with a very different tone, one now of respect, but I did not answer or return her call. I thought it would be better to move on than to put both of us in a very awkward situation. A friend told me about a job loading trucks at night at UPS, which I took. Between going to classes, studying, and working nights, I spent what little time I had left researching residency programs.

● ● ● ●

I filled out more than a hundred residency program applications in the tiny attic room I rented from the elderly woman near the University of Washington Medical Center. I basically sent one to every pathology program I could find. When I did not receive any responses, I began sending applications to internal medicine and family practice programs as well. After sending out a very large number of applications, I came home one day and found a letter waiting for me. It came from one of the top hospitals in Seattle. I ripped the envelope open, excitedly expecting good news inside. Instead I found a handwritten note attached to my application package just as I had sent it. The note read, "You are not as competitive as the doctors who work here. Please go back to Africa where you came from. You are not good enough to work here, and we don't think you ever will be." I dropped the letter and wept.

Out of the more than a hundred applications I sent out, I only received two invitations to fly out to a program and interview for one of their positions. I flew to Massachusetts for one interview and to New York City for the other. The flights drained all my savings. I started looking for a better job and found one in a local nursing home. I went to work as a nurse's aide. Most days I started work around 4:00 p.m. or 9:00 p.m.

and worked until 12:00 a.m. or 5:00 a.m., respectively. The bus ride to and from work took about two hours each way, which was when I slept. I didn't have much choice. This was the only way I was going to survive.

Most of the patients with whom I worked at the nursing home suffered from dementia, and most were women. My duties included delivering their meals, giving them baths, cleaning them up when they soiled themselves, changing their diapers, and dressing and undressing them, as well as helping them walk around or pushing them in their wheelchairs. I put them to bed at night and read to them or even sang them to sleep. Like I said, most suffered from some form of dementia.

I had one lovely patient who was more on the obese side and was not in her right mind. Every time I walked into her room, she said to me, "Nigger, you don't belong here. You get away from me. Don't you dare touch me." I passed it off as the dementia talking. She didn't know what she was saying. I had to do my job, so I did it. More than once she became very agitated by my presence. Several times she spat at me. I just laughed it off. My supervisor saw what was going on and was shocked by it. "It doesn't bother me," I said. "She's just a poor, demented woman. I don't know how I might act if I were in her place."

• • • •

Match Day came in March 1995. This is the day when residency programs announce who they are inviting to come join them. The whole match process is rather odd. At every other stage of higher education, you choose where you want to go. You choose your college—as long as they accept you. The same is true of graduate programs and professional programs like law school and med school. However, for residency you go out and interview with as many programs as give you the opportunity. You then list them in order of your preference. The programs then decide who is going where. You have very little say in the matter. If you do not like where you have matched, you have few options for going elsewhere.

Since I had only interviewed in two places, I didn't care which one chose me as long as one did. That would have been my attitude even if I had had a hundred interviews. I just wanted to match somewhere. Anywhere.

But I did not. No offer came from Massachusetts or New York. I only had one option. As soon as my one-year visiting scholar program ended, I was going to have to get on a plane and fly back to Nigeria. My visa was going to expire, and the United States had no reason to renew it.

After learning of my failure to match, I went back to my small attic room, disappointed and angry. I wasn't just disappointed and angry in a general sense. All of my frustrations were aimed at one individual—the One I blamed for the mess in which I now found myself. I was angry at God and I was not shy about telling Him so. "How could You lead me so far, only to leave me in the middle of the sea to drown?" I asked Him. "If I knew this was what You were going to do to me, I never would have left home to begin with. I never would have worked so hard to come to America." I guess you can call this prayer, since I was talking to God. If so, you can say I prayed for most of the night. I unloaded on Him. "All of this was a sham, a cruel joke You have played on me," I prayed, "I wish You would have just left me alone and that You would leave me alone now." At one point after expressing my disappointed frustrations with God, I collapsed into tears.

I wanted to go to sleep, but I could not. Emotionally spent, I rolled over on my bed and looked at the clock, which read 3:00. I felt so alone and lonely and hopeless in that tiny attic room. Finally, my eyelids started to feel heavy, as if sleep was going to take me after all. In that moment of finally feeling like rest was near, my heart turned loose of its last piece of bitterness. I whispered in the dark, "Oh, God, I do believe and trust You and love You. All things are possible with You, and You can make a way if You choose. All things were made by You and for You and exist in You. In the name of Jesus, I confess that all things are possible in You." I still felt the hopelessness and doubt and despair, but one thing I knew above all others: I could not turn away from my God. I did not know what He had planned for me, but I trusted Him with my life.

I drifted off to sleep, planning to stay in bed all the next day and maybe even the day after that. With that, I passed out.

The phone started ringing at 6:30 a.m. I slapped at it like it was the alarm and I was trying to reach the snooze button. I woke up enough to pick up the phone and say hello. On the other end, I heard a deep, baritone voice with a Mexican accent. "Dr. Omalu?" he asked.

"Yes, this is Dr. Bennet Omalu," I said, now more awake.

"This is Dr. Carlos Navarro, professor of pathology at the College of Physicians and Surgeons at Colombia University and director of the residency program at Harlem Hospital Center. I apologize for calling so early. I hope I didn't wake you."

"No, no, no, it's not too early," I lied.

"I'll get right to the point. Have you already matched with a program?" Dr. Navarro asked.

"No, I haven't."

"Good. We did not offer you one of the two positions we had open. However, one of the doctors to whom we offered it has turned us down."

"Okay," I said.

"We would like tentatively to offer the position to you."

I could hardly believe my ears. "Okay," I said, almost in shock. "What do I need to do?"

"Would it be possible for you to come back to New York City tomorrow and meet with the director of the department of pathology? She was not available when you interviewed with us the first time."

"I would love to do that, but . . ." I hesitated. "To be honest with you, Dr. Navarro, I cannot spend so much money on a last-minute flight to New York and then have you not accept me."

Dr. Navarro gave me a reassuring laugh. "I understand," he said. "Now, while I cannot guarantee that you will be offered the position, I can say there is a 95 percent chance the spot is yours."

"That's good enough for me," I said. "I will be there first thing tomorrow morning."

After I hung up the phone, I went to the bank to check my balance.

I had about $1,500 in my account because I had just been paid by the nursing home. I took $1,200 and bought a red-eye ticket to New York. Fifteen hours later, I was at LaGuardia Airport, dressed in my best suit with $100 in my pocket. I took the subway train to Harlem Hospital for my meeting with the pathology department director. After the meeting, I rode the train back to LaGuardia. My flight didn't leave until early the next morning, but I did not have the money to stay in a hotel that night. Instead I found a spot on the floor in the check-in lounge and slept there in my suit. About ten other people joined me there, although I was the only one wearing a tie.

A day or so after I arrived back home in Seattle, Dr. Navarro called. "Dr. Omalu, Bennet, I am delighted to tell you that we would like to offer you a spot in our residency program starting this summer."

Of course I accepted.

After I hung up the phone, I thought back to that dark night when I had lost all hope and nearly lost my faith. The Bible says, "Faith is the realization of what is hoped for and evidence of things not seen."[1] When I allowed my frustration to boil over into anger at God, I could only see what was in front of me. That was why doubt came. I wanted to give up in the face of difficulty. The Lord seemed to whisper to me in that moment, "Bennet, life is a struggle. Christ struggled, but He never wavered. So you too must not give up or give in for the purpose I have for you. You have to continue fighting the good fight and running the good race. You cannot tire until you take your last breath. You will rest eternally when I call you home." Those were my last thoughts that night when I fell asleep, and now God had shown me how faithful He truly is.

I hoped to match with *any* residency program. God wanted me in Harlem in a program connected to an Ivy League school. Just because I did not initially match with them was not a problem for God. I had lost sight of the evidence of things not seen. I prayed I would not make that mistake again.

Chapter Eight

Land of Contradictions

When I decided to go public with what I discovered in my autopsy of Mike Webster in 2002, I naively believed America and the National Football League would welcome my findings. Growing up in Nigeria and looking longingly at America from afar, I believed the United States to be free of corruption and hidden agendas. I thought it to be a place where people love and value truth to such a degree that they would want to know the truth about what the game of football can do to those who play it. I wanted to announce the Mike Webster case on the home turf of the NFL because I believed my discovery was good for football and would make it a better, safer game more in line with the trends of American society in the twenty-first century. Since football is America's game, I thought what would be good for football would be good for America and good for the humanity in us all.

But my findings were not welcomed by the NFL, nor were they embraced by American society as a whole. As you will read more about later, the NFL tried to destroy my career. By the time they were finished with me, I had lost nearly everything I held dear. Their attacks were swift and severe, as they demanded an immediate retraction after my first paper on Chronic Traumatic Encephalopathy (CTE) was published in *Neurosurgery* (the official journal of the Congress of Neurological Surgeons) in 2005. Much of the latter half of this book will chronicle my ensuing battle with the NFL—a battle that in some ways continues to this day.

Looking back, I now know I should not have been surprised at the NFL's response. After all, claiming that football caused life-altering, and ultimately life-shortening, brain damage threatens the football industry's long-term viability. As one of the doctors connected to the NFL said to me in a private meeting, if just 10 percent of the mothers in America stopped allowing their sons to play the game, the sport is finished. He said this to me more than a decade ago. I believe his words to be prophetic.

The doctor may be correct in the long term, but what has surprised me in the fifteen years since I discovered CTE is how football's popularity as a spectator sport remains, in spite of negative headlines concerning football and brain disease. Not even the suicide of one of the most popular players to ever play the game, Junior Seau—a suicide prompted by the depression and behavior changes caused by CTE—has dented football's popularity. The American public holds up football stars as heroes. Yet when one of those heroes dies as a direct result of playing the game, the public simply shrugs and keeps watching. For proof you need look no further than the ratings for the Super Bowl, an event that has become an American holiday. The last nine Super Bowls account for nine of the ten highest-rated television broadcasts of all time.

That leads me to wonder: *How can Americans idolize football players, yet seem to care so little about the toll the game takes upon their heroes?* It seems like such a contradiction. Yet as I learned after moving to Harlem in June 1995, America is a land of contradictions. I am truly an American, because my time in Harlem revealed the contradictions deep inside of me as well.

• • • •

When I landed at LaGuardia Airport after moving from Seattle to New York, everything I owned in this world fit into one suitcase. Even though I had lived in America for a year, I still knew very little about how to conduct myself in my new country. I stepped out of the airport as the sun started to set and tried to hail a cab. One or two cabbies asked me where I wanted to go. "Harlem," I said. I did not understand how odd it looked to these cabbies that a young black man wanted to go to Harlem after dark. No one volunteered to take me.

Every cab passed me by and picked up the next person in line until finally a cab driven by an older man with a thick Indian accent agreed to take me. I handed him the address, and we took off. I stared out the window at my new hometown as we sped down the freeway and zipped across bridges. The huge buildings mesmerized me. I had never seen anything like them in my life. The city changed when we exited the freeway and wound through the neighborhoods leading to Harlem. I noticed that the closer we got to Harlem, the more the cab had to dodge holes in the streets. The buildings appeared more dilapidated. At first I thought this might be because the streets were darker, with fewer working streetlights, but in the weeks that followed, I discovered the buildings were just run-down.

Finally, the cab pulled up in front of a two-story brick building. "This is it," he said.

I looked out at an old building behind the hospital on a poorly lit street filled with all types of debris. It looked like the building had seen better days and was likely in need of some serious renovation and retouching of the brick. "*This?*" I asked.

"Yes, this is the address you gave me," the cabbie said, more than a little annoyed.

"Okay, thank you," I said. "How much is the fare?"

He told me the amount. I paid him exactly what he told me. The cabbie looked at the money and glared at me. "Why, you cheap . . ." he said, unleashing a string of names and curses as he put the car in gear and sped away. I had no idea why he was angry. A few months passed before I discovered that you are supposed to tip taxi drivers and waiters and waitresses.

In spite of my rocky introduction to the city, I soon fell in love with New York. Never before in my life had I encountered such an amazing mix of people from all types of backgrounds, religions, ethnicities, and creeds. In Nigeria, people were divided by tribe, with distinct tribal dialects and languages. However, no matter the tribe, everyone looked very similar to one another. But New York was a melting pot of people from all over the world. I had never seen such a mix in my life. And the languages! The first time I heard someone speaking Spanish I thought they were singing as they spoke. It was beautiful, as were the Hispanic women I met at the hospital.

I so loved the blend of people and cultures in New York that I used to go out on Sundays to a busy part of Manhattan just to people-watch. I found a restaurant with an outside patio, ordered something to eat and drink, and soaked in everything around me. The diversity gave me great joy and reaffirmed to me our common humanity. Black and white, Hispanic, Asian, Native American, Jew and Gentile—we are all a very beautiful people, and all were here in New York, in America. I could hear the words of the Declaration of Independence ringing in my ears. Surely this was the place where the truth that all people are created equal had finally come to light.

However, the wonder I felt in Manhattan eventually gave way to a stark reality. For nine months I lived in a dormitory maintained by the hospital for single residents like me. Life in the dorm got old fast. I started looking for an apartment in Midtown Manhattan near the areas where I liked to go to people-watch. I walked up and down the streets and took note of apartments with vacancies. I called several, but for some reason, whenever they heard my accent, they said they no longer had a vacancy. Undeterred, I started going to the apartments to inquire in person. After all, I was a doctor, albeit still a resident. I thought if I talked to the apartment managers, I could dispel any fears they might have about my ability to pay. But going to the apartments in person was even worse. I hardly had a chance to open my mouth before being told there were no vacancies.

After having door after door closed to me, I decided to conduct an experiment. I told a Jewish friend what had happened, and he went with me the next time I went apartment hunting. First, I went into the rental office and asked about their advertised vacancies. "We don't have any vacancies," the office manager said bluntly. Ten minutes later, my friend went into the same office and asked the same question. "Of course, we have several. In fact, you can move in this week if you like," he was told. On our way back to Harlem, my friend told me I should file a complaint with the housing commission, but I brushed his suggestion aside. If I filed a complaint every time a taxi driver refused to pick me up or a bank teller questioned the legitimacy of one of my checks, I would go crazy. New York may have been a melting pot, but it was still a city with deep racial divides.

Eventually, I moved to the nearby town of Lodi, New Jersey, and commuted to the hospital in a new Volkswagen Jetta I leased. This was my first major purchase in America. However, the toll fees nearly left me broke, along with the cost of parking and insurance. I didn't make much as a resident physician, and a significant amount of what I made went back to Nigeria to help support my family. So I returned my car and moved to a studio apartment in the heart of Harlem on 149th Street. For four years I walked back and forth from my apartment to the hospital. That's when I came face-to-face with the immense hopelessness, deprivation, and apathy that came with the extreme poverty I saw every day. I talked with very strong people who had been bruised and battered by a system they felt locked them out of any meaningful opportunity. The neighborhood reaffirmed the same message. Unlike the bright, clean, well-lit neighborhoods of Midtown, these streets were dirty and dark. Even though the two places were separated by only a few miles, traveling from one to the other made me feel like I had stepped onto a different continent.

Still, I held out hope in the American dream. I believed that by hard work and determination, anyone could find their way here. One day while working at the hospital, I tried to encourage one of the young black men working in the department to further his education and not to limit himself in his expectations. He looked at me with tears in his eyes and said, "You don't get it, man. You're lucky because you weren't born here."

His words took me aback. "What do you mean?" I asked.

"If you had been born here in this neighborhood, you never would have become a doctor. From day one, people would have had you pegged. You never would have had the chance to become a doctor. Never."

Twenty years later as I write these words, I can still see the look in his eyes. This wasn't just about racism. He spoke of a reality, where your slot in society is already set from the day of your birth before you do anything. I know there are exceptions and that opportunities can be found, but the core of what he said to me has not changed. That's one of the great contradictions of America. All people are created equal, yet without even realizing it, we prejudge some as less, all because of the color of their skin or the neighborhood where they grow up or both. This is a great land, the freest nation on earth and in history, yet it is still a land of contradictions. The problem does not lie in America but in the human heart, as I learned in a very personal way.

• • • •

In a way I am surprised that I had any time to observe anything outside of the Harlem Hospital Center. My residency training filled nearly every waking hour of my life. Like all residency programs in every field of medicine, mine consisted of multiple four- to twelve-week rotations where I focused on different areas of both anatomic pathology (AP) and clinical pathology (CP). Pathology itself is the specialty that deals with the causes and nature of disease. Anatomic pathologists investigate the effects of disease on the human body through autopsies and microscopic examination of tissues, cells, and other specimens. My AP rotations included autopsy pathology, forensic pathology, cytopathology, surgical pathology, and a couple more.

Clinical pathology focuses more on the diagnostic interpretation of laboratory tests. These rotations included clinical chemistry, immunology, medical microbiology, and molecular diagnostics, as well as several more areas. Both specialties meant I spent a lot of time peering through a microscope searching for answers hidden in the cells in front of me.

When some of my friends back in Nigeria heard what I was doing, they told me I was wasting my time and talents. But I disagreed. Pathology fed my natural curiosity. I found I could spend hours doing research, and the time passed quickly without my even noticing it.

I faced a challenge, however, right out of the gate. My very first rotation of my first week of my first year of residency was autopsy pathology. Back in medical school, I had worked with cadavers, but this was very different. Now my task was not to learn and understand human anatomy. No, I had to discover the reason the person in front of me had died.

My first autopsy began before I even saw my first "patient." One of the technical support staff brought a file of medical records to my desk for me to study before the actual autopsy began. This was in 1995—in the dark days when the AIDS epidemic still ran through New York City and all the major cities in the United States. According to his records, the man I was to examine had full-blown AIDS, which had taken his life. However, the question I had to answer was how.

The autopsy suite was located in the basement of the hospital adjacent to the morgue. When I arrived shortly after 11:00 a.m., the body was lying on an examination table, waiting for me. I changed into my green scrubs and suited up in all the protective gear to protect me from the infectious diseases that had taken this man's life. Returning to the autopsy room, I found the chief resident was there to guide me through the autopsy protocol and assist me if I needed any help.

I must confess that I needed help right from the moment I walked into the room. The smell of death permeated everything. The smell only grew worse when the body's thoracic and abdominal cavities were opened. "Let's get started," the chief resident said. He pointed to where I was to make the first incision with the scalpel. I hesitated for a moment as I stared at the body lying in front of me. I had never seen such an emaciated individual. He looked like a scary masquerade of a human body, like a skeleton that had slipped on a suit of skin. Lesions covered the body, including purple Kaposi sarcoma welts. At that moment I felt like throwing off my protective gear and running out of the room and off to nowhere, never to look back. A lump rose in my throat. The sides of my cheeks squeezed in. I knew I was going to throw up at any moment. The chief resident didn't notice—or if he did, he didn't care. He was too busy chatting away and laughing with one of the autopsy technicians. The shock at seeing this sight had long since worn off for him.

I stared down at the body. I knew I could not run away. My journey from Nigeria to Seattle had brought me here. If I were to quit, all I had worked for would be lost. Touching this body, cutting into it, and spending time with it was my only choice. Honestly, I felt like a condemned man.

Pushing back my nausea, I started the physical examination by ticking off the boxes on the autopsy worksheet. "Hair, black," I said. "Eyes, brown. The body is in poor condition with multiple lesions. Subject appears to be malnourished."

As I ticked off the boxes, a strange feeling came over me. I looked down at the body, but I did not see just a body in front of me; I saw an individual. This man was a human being just like me. He had been someone's brother, someone's cousin, a boyfriend or husband, a mother and father's son. The emaciated condition of the body that had repulsed me now called to me. This man lying in front of me had been the victim of a disease that had caused him to die far too soon. I looked into his face. I saw myself there. He could have been me, and I could have been him. In that moment, the two of us became one.

Death strips away all dignity, just as this man had been stripped and laid bare before me. As I made my first incision into his body, I felt my job, my calling, was to restore his dignity by discovering the true reason for his death. In this way I felt I was preparing him for his transition into heaven. The autopsy then became a spiritual experience for me. I was treading on holy ground. The smell did not matter anymore. I methodically and systematically took sections of his organs and tissues, like I was painting a masterpiece. Before I knew it, the autopsy was finished. Two hours flew by as if only a few minutes had passed.

I removed my scrubs and went to my desk to record all my notes from the procedure. I meticulously described what I had observed into an autopsy narrative. The head of the program, the man who brought me to Harlem, Dr. Carlos Navarro, went through my work with me and asked me questions. At the end, he patted me on the shoulder. "Good job, Bennet," he said. "Very good job." Several weeks later the two of us examined the microscopic sections of the man's tissues, which had now been stained and prepared for further examination. These slides were beautiful and different. Dr. Navarro guided me through the derivative thinking and analysis of each slide and led me through the process of differential diagnosis. We determined the man died of acute respiratory failure due to a type of pneumonia that only strikes immunosuppressed people like victims of AIDS.

When we finished our analysis, I finalized my autopsy report and enumerated all the pathologic findings. I signed the report, as did Dr. Navarro. This was his final stamp of approval of a job well done. My first autopsy was my first step into learning the language of the dead. I was learning to listen to them and to ask them the right questions. With time, I became so in tune with the dead that when I learned how someone died, I could tell you how he or she lived. It was truly a spiritual experience.

. . . .

Unfortunately, the deep spiritual moments were rare during my residency. My schedule was brutal, and I felt very much alone. All my family was on the other side of the world, and calling them was very expensive. The depression I experienced in medical school reemerged. Rather than withdraw, I went in the other direction. While at the hospital, I poured myself into my duties and worked like a maniac. When I was off duty, I partied. I was wild and smoked and drank. Sex became something I looked for in women as I went to the clubs. It seemed like there was no end to my appetites. It was like I was addicted. I simply went crazy.

At the same time, I kept going to church and praying. I felt like a prodigal son. The contradiction of my life tore me up inside. On Saturday nights, I went out and partied as hard as I could. On Sundays, I went to church and pleaded for forgiveness, while promising God I was going to change my ways. One Sunday in particular, I knelt at the Communion altar rail, making promises to God. When I looked up, the woman serving Communion winked at me. We had been together the night before in her apartment. That afternoon, we were back there, doing what men and women do in those settings. I was a mess.

Then one day, I began to feel weak. I had also begun to lose weight, and I had zero energy. Some days I barely had the strength to get out of bed. I felt for lymph nodes in my armpits, only to discover they were swollen. I recognized the symptoms. I'd read the same symptoms in medical charts at least once a week during my autopsy rotations when a victim of AIDS came across my table. I immediately made an appointment with a doctor in Manhattan, who confirmed my fears. "You may well have contracted HIV," he told me. "We will have to do a blood test to tell for sure."

That was a Friday afternoon. What followed was the longest, darkest weekend of my life. On Saturday, I tried to drink and smoke away my pain. On Sunday, I got up and went to church and pleaded with God to save me. On Monday morning, I called in sick to work. I could not go in and face more death, not with a possible death sentence hanging over my head. My mind went back to that first autopsy. *He could be me, and I could be him*, I had thought at the time. Now these thoughts haunted me.

I called my sister Winny and told her what was going on. "If the test comes back positive, I will probably kill myself rather than sit around and wait to die in some horrible way," I told her.

"Don't worry, Bene," Winny said. "We offered you up to God before you left Nigeria. He will take care of you." She then pleaded with me to come back home to Nigeria if the test came back positive. "You will not suffer alone," she said.

"Okay," I said, but I didn't really mean it. To be honest, I could not contemplate a future that dark.

Later that afternoon, my phone rang. A lovely feminine voice on the other end asked, "Is this Bennet—Bennet Omalu?"

I swallowed hard. "Yes," I replied.

"I called to give you your HIV status result. The physician left a note that we should call you."

I almost collapsed in fear when I heard that.

"Your test came back negative," she said. "However, other tests show that you may have infectious mononucleosis. We need you to come back to see the doctor this week. Does tomorrow work for you?"

I was so relieved by the good news that I nearly shouted, "Yes, tomorrow, I will be there!" When I hung up the phone, I collapsed back onto my bed, relieved and grateful. I poured out my thanks to God for sparing my life.

One might think that after such a close brush with death, I would immediately change my behavior. However, within a matter of days, I was right back where I was before, working like a maniac and partying like a maniac. Thankfully, God was merciful, even as I know He grew tired of my contradiction of a life. At one point, I discovered I was impotent. That didn't immediately cause me to change my ways. I went to see a urologist, who found nothing physically wrong with me. He sent me to a psychiatrist. My sessions with him yielded no answers. The problem persisted.

One morning during a time of prayer, the answer came to me. God had done this to me to put an end to my contradictory lifestyle. He had too much in store for me to throw it away, as I tried to do during my time in New York. Once I accepted His plan, I was ready for the next step along His path. My struggles with temptation did not immediately end. Do they ever? However, I found myself filled with thanks to God that He still loved me in spite of myself and in spite of my contradictions. His mercy gave me hope for myself, and for my adopted home.

Chapter Nine

A Bold Gamble

By my second year of residency, I knew I wanted to specialize in forensic pathology. The reason circled back to the feelings I had during my first years of clinical medicine in Nigeria. Forensic pathology placed me as far away as possible from living, breathing patients, while still allowing me to practice medicine. However, there was more to my decision than that. While no one wants to spend their career surrounded by death, I found a deep sense of satisfaction in bringing dignity to those upon whom I worked. I became like a servant who prepared his master for the great beyond by the cleansing of the autopsy, as though this was a vital step in the transition from earth to heaven.

I was also good at it.

Dr. Carlos Navarro deserves the credit for that. He became a mentor and the father I did not have in New York. I worked alongside him, and he guided me and the other residents through every step of derivative tissue diagnosis. When I had the privilege of working with him on an autopsy, I felt like I was watching Michael Jordan doing his thing on a basketball court or Michael Jackson moonwalking across a stage. Dr. Navarro wasn't just a skilled pathologist; he applied a level of artistry and perfection that made me want to develop my skills to be the best I could possibly be. Without a doubt, he was the single most influential person in my life in preparing me for the career God had for me. He instilled in me the love for the autopsy and shaped me into the doctor and man I am today. During my residency period, I did not take any vacation days. I felt I had a lot of ground to make up, since I was twenty-six by the time I came to America. Dr. Navarro kindly supported me with whatever I needed to succeed. If this sounds like I am gushing about my mentor, I am. I cannot overemphasize the impact he had upon my life.

By my third year, I knew I needed to figure out my next move. If I was to become a forensic pathologist, I needed to be accepted into a fellowship program after my residency. That is the way of medicine. Medical school prepares you for a career in medicine in a very general way. You study all aspects of medicine and spend four years doing rotations in nearly every field—from anatomy to physiology, surgery to internal medicine to obstetrics and gynecology, etc. Throughout the three to seven years of residency, you focus on one field of medicine, but also in a more general way. Finally, you hone your skills during one- to four-year fellowships in one or more subspecialties.

The fact that I was an international medical graduate put me at a disadvantage. Fellowships are highly competitive. In those days, most programs were less likely to give me the benefit of a doubt without knowing who I was. But how could they get to know me? I needed some sort of personal touch to overcome the natural barrier of my background. If I did not secure a fellowship, my visa status would be revoked, and I would have to leave the United States. For me, that was not an option.

I began to pray and ask God to guide me and open the right doors for me. Just like the answer to my prayers years earlier in Nigeria, God's answer came in the form of a letter.

One morning when I walked into the Harlem Hospital Center, Dr. Navarro greeted me with an envelope in his hand. "I think this is something you should pursue," he said.

I opened the letter, which came from Dr. Abdulrezak Shakir, the program director for the fellowship training program in forensic pathology in Allegheny County, Pennsylvania. After reading the letter, I came up with a plan. Rather than just apply to the program, I decided to send a letter to Dr. Shakir, asking him if I could visit their office for a one-month, self-financed externship without pay. I believed this would give me a chance to prove myself while also giving them an opportunity to get to know me and my skills. The gesture may have been out of the box, but I needed to do something to stand out from all the other applicants. Dr. Navarro also wrote a letter of recommendation for me.

Several weeks went by. Finally I heard back from Dr. Shakir, telling me that my externship had been approved. I just needed to let them know when I was available to do it. My spirits soared. I went to Dr. Navarro and explained the situation to him. Since I had never taken any of my allotted vacation time, Dr. Navarro modified my schedule to give me the entire month of October 1998 off. With that, I packed my bags, rented a car, bought a map, and headed west on Interstate 80, bound for Pittsburgh.

The eight-hour drive from New York to Pittsburgh gave me my first real chance to see America. Even though I had lived on both coasts, I had seen very little of the country outside of Seattle and New York. Driving down Interstate 80, with Rod Stewart blaring from the car's CD player, I marveled at the beauty of the Pennsylvania mountains, hills, and plains. The leaves had started to turn, which set the hills ablaze with color. Because Nigeria sits so close to the equator, it does not experience dramatic changes of season. Trees stay green all year round. But not here, not in the mountains of Pennsylvania. It was as though God had pulled out His watercolor set and painted a masterpiece for me to enjoy.

I got to Pittsburgh around 7:00 p.m. on a Sunday. It was a dark and rainy evening. I found the coroner's office on Fourth Avenue in downtown Pittsburgh. They were expecting me. One of the death investigators took me over to the Renaissance Hotel, where I spent my first night. Later, I moved to an extended-stay hotel, where the rent was much cheaper.

Early Monday morning, I reported for duty at the Allegheny County coroner's office. A staff member greeted me and showed me around briefly. "You can change in there into your scrubs," she said, pointing to the staff locker room. "The autopsy room is right over there. Dr. Rozin is waiting for you." Dr. Leon Rozin was the chief forensic pathologist and was on duty that day.

"Okay, thank you," I replied.

I quickly changed into green scrubs and went into the autopsy suite. "You Omalu?" Dr. Rozin said to me as I walked in.

"Yes, sir. Bennet Omalu," I said, extending my hand.

"Yeah, good to meet you," Dr. Rozin said politely but not enthusiastically. He pointed over to the table closest to the exit door. A young white male lay on the table. "That one's yours. The instruments are already laid out for you," he said. "You can handle this by yourself, right?"

I hoped the expression on my face didn't give me away. I lied and said, "Yes. Of course. Thank you." In truth I had never performed an autopsy all by myself. An attending physician always supervised me at Harlem Hospital Center. Nor had I ever performed a forensic autopsy, where the cause of death is completely unknown. For most cases in the hospital autopsies I had performed, we already knew generally why and how a person died. Those autopsies studied the body for differential diagnoses, quality assurance, and academic purposes. Now I had to determine the cause of a sudden and unexpected death.

Dr. Rozin turned and walked to another table in the suite. Slowly, I walked over to the autopsy table. A technician handed me a file with the case narrative. "White male . . . twenty years old . . . found dead in his bed in the morning . . . no abrasions or lacerations on the body . . . no other signs of foul play." I glanced around the autopsy suite. Everyone was busy doing what they were supposed to be doing, and no one paid any attention to me. If I had turned around and called over to Dr. Rozin and told him I could not do this, my chances of a fellowship would end right there. Nor could I call out to anyone else in the room for help. These were all strangers to me—strangers who had their hands full with their own work.

I looked down at the face of the young man lying in front of me. He seemed so young. As I stared at him, a revelation came to me. *He* knew how he had died. All I needed was for him to tell me. I patted the young man on the shoulder and called out his name. Very softly I said, "Please help me. Show me why you died. I am afraid, and I have never done this before. But I don't want to let myself down, and I don't want to let you down. Help me, please."

My fears suddenly evaporated. I felt that the spirit of the young man was in the room. You can think what you may of that statement, but I am telling you what I experienced in that moment. Confidence filled my soul as I took a scalpel and made the first incision. Slowly, methodically, I checked each vital organ, weighing them, examining them closely. Given the facts of the case, I went through and eliminated every possible reason for a sudden death. His heart was strong and healthy, as were his lungs. I found no signs of a stroke in his brain. Nothing looked out of the ordinary. Given his physical condition, this young man should have been anywhere other than my autopsy table.

After two hours, I was done. The autopsy technician packed the dissected organs back into the body cavities and stitched him closed. I put my notes together and went to find Dr. Rozin. "I can find no physical cause of death. Everything checks out perfectly. I believe he died from a drug overdose, but we will have to wait for the toxicology reports to come back to know for sure," I said.

"Very nice work, Dr. Omalu," Dr. Rozin said to me. "I'm impressed."

"Thank you," I said. I then walked back over to the young man on the table. "Thank you," I said very softly. "Thank you so much for what you have done for me. I hope this gives you peace."

When the toxicology report came back, it confirmed my diagnosis.

Over the course of the next month, I threw myself headlong into my work. Every morning, I tried to be the first doctor to arrive at the office and the last to leave. No matter what I was asked to do, I did it without griping or complaining. Following the example of my mentor, Dr. Navarro, I tried to elevate my performance each and every day, to improve my skills and not be satisfied with good enough. I got to know the other people in the office and established good relationships with them. The longer I was there, the more I wanted to come back and work here. I liked this place.

I also began to do some research into the Allegheny County coroner's office. Dr. Cyril Wecht, the coroner, was, I learned, basically a rock star in the world of forensic medicine. He first became a public figure in the 1960s, when he poked holes in the Warren Commission's findings that President Kennedy had been killed by a single shooter. In his assessment, the prevailing global forensic scenario and medical evidence simply did not support that. When I read of his connection to the JFK investigation, a bell went off in my head. I had heard his name years before when I watched a documentary about President Kennedy while I still lived in Nigeria. After making a name for himself with his response to the Warren Commission report, Dr. Wecht was part of some of the biggest cases in America, including investigating the deaths of Robert Kennedy, JonBenét Ramsey, and the victims of the Manson family murders. He'd penned bestselling books about famous and infamous murder cases and was brought in as a forensic expert by attorneys like F. Lee Bailey. The more I discovered about Dr. Wecht, the more I realized that working in his office was the chance of a lifetime for an aspiring forensic pathologist like myself.

I met Dr. Wecht for the first time on the first day of my externship when he took me and the other pathologists in the office out for lunch. He immediately struck me as a man who was different from others. Forthright and no-nonsense, with an assertive persona, Cyril Wecht spoke his mind and was not afraid to go against the tide of popular opinion when he believed he was right. And when he believed he was right, I found he usually *was* right. His jovial loquaciousness struck some as abrasive. Me—I found it refreshing. He had a good, transparent, and sincere heart, while also doing his work at a level few people have ever attained.

During my first meeting with Dr. Wecht, he turned to me and asked, "So how did you get Harlem Hospital Center to pay for this externship? If they're like our office, money is always tight."

"The hospital isn't paying for my time here," I answered.

Dr. Wecht looked at me with surprise. "Then who is? I don't recall signing off on a grant for you."

"I'm paying for this myself," I said.

"You're what?" he said, with more than a little shock in his voice.

"I knew this was a once-in-a-lifetime opportunity, so I am paying for everything myself," I said.

Dr. Wecht smiled. "You won't mind if I pick up our lunch tab, then?" he said jokingly.

I laughed. "No, not at all. Thank you." From that moment forward, I think I had a special place in Dr. Wecht's heart. In me he saw someone just as driven to succeed as he was. And in him I saw someone after whom I knew I should pattern myself.

I came to Pittsburgh to audition for a fellowship, but I also came here to learn. Early on, I learned to take Dr. Wecht's advice. Once while making a presentation on a case to him and several other people in his office, I humbly offered my opinion as to what had happened to the deceased person. I used words like *may* and *might* and *possibly* throughout my presentation. Dr. Wecht stopped me in the middle and said, "Bennet, Bennet, Bennet, you are now in America. I know you were raised in a former British colony and in the old British way, where being meek is regarded as strength. But not in America. You have to be assertive, speak out confidently, and be bold and arrogant if need be. Americans respect that. If you come across as meek in America, some people will want to run right over you."

He did not have to tell me twice. I edited out such words from all future presentations. When I knew, I said it boldly. If I did not know, I said that as well.

At the end of my month in Pittsburgh, Dr. Wecht asked me to come see him in his office. "Bennet, the fellowship position is yours if you want it," he said. "We'd be honored to have you join us here in Pittsburgh."

I fought back tears, smiled, and said, "Thank you. Yes, sir, I would love to join you here. Thank you for offering the position to me."

At that moment, I had no idea what was ahead of me in Pittsburgh, nor how this externship would change the course of my entire life. For now, I was simply grateful for the opportunity.

• • • •

Before I could begin my work in Pittsburgh, I had to finish my residency in Harlem. The anatomic and clinical pathology residency program was five years when I started in 1995. I applied to the American Board of Pathology to reduce my five-year training to four. Given the progress I'd made and the position waiting for me in Pennsylvania, I did not believe I needed the fifth year. In my application letter, I included academic justifications, along with a list of professional accomplishments to support my request. Dr. Navarro penned a support letter for me. A short time after submitting my request, the board sent me an approval letter.

I spent my final months in New York learning all I could from Dr. Navarro and the rest of the staff at Harlem Hospital Center. With the fellowship in hand, I was able to focus more clearly on exactly those skills I needed to hone to be ready for my work at the Allegheny County coroner's office, which was converted into a medical examiner's office in 2005.

At the end of the academic year, I gave away most of the possessions I had acquired while living in my Harlem studio apartment. I loaded what was left into another rental car and set sail on Interstate 80 on a warm June 1999 morning. Once I left the city, I pulled the car onto the shoulder of the freeway, stepped out of the car, and took one long, last look at the city that had given me so much. The twin towers stood as majestic as ever over the New York skyline. "Thank you, New York," I said. "I hope Pittsburgh will give me what you have given me." I let out a long sigh, got back in my car, and pulled back out on the highway headed southwest.

Teddy Pendergrass filled the car. As the highway rolled beneath my car, I felt very optimistic about the future. New York had been good to me, but I knew it was time to leave the hustle and bustle of the city behind. This move was therapeutic for me. Over the previous four years, I had proved that I belonged here. I had completed a program through the College of Physicians and Surgeons of Columbia University, an Ivy

League school, and had been accepted into a fellowship program supervised by one of the leading forensic pathologists in the United States, if not the world. However, these past four years had left me mentally, emotionally, and spiritually exhausted. I hoped the more laid-back and less cosmopolitan Pittsburgh would be exactly what I needed to get my mind back. Either way, I could not wait to get there and get on with the next chapter of my life.

Chapter Ten

Finding Myself

When I graduated from medical school, all I really wanted to be was myself. That seems like an easy thing to do, but it is very difficult when you do not really know who you are. Many of the decisions about which I have written thus far were more about who I did *not* want to be than about who I am. I went to medical school at the insistence of my father, but I did *not* want to be a doctor. When an opportunity came to go to Seattle to study the epidemiology of cancer, I took it, not because I wanted to study the epidemiology of cancer, but because it brought me to America.

Once I was in America, I completed a pathology residency, not out of a sense of calling or because I found fulfillment as a pathologist. I was better suited for work in a pathology lab than in a clinic with one live patient after another. After my four years of residency, I pursued a fellowship in forensic pathology primarily because it took me even further away from clinical medicine while allowing me to remain in America. Growing up in Nigeria, I never dreamed of spending my life conducting autopsies and investigating causes of death. Even today, I have friends from back home who say to me, "Bennet, how can you spend your life surrounded by death? That doesn't seem like you."

Working with the dead did *not* seem like me, but then again, nothing really seemed like me because I did not know who I was. In the movie *Concussion*, Will Smith, playing me, says, "In America, you must be the best version of yourself. If you do not know what that is, you pick something and fake it." I did not know what the best version of me might be—or any version of me—so I picked someone, and I faked it. Faking it may sound like the opposite of being oneself, but that was not the case for me. Long before I ever came to America, I was attracted to this nation by her creativity and the perfection I found in American music. Watching American music videos on satellite television as a boy in Nigeria, I promised myself that whatever I did in life, I would strive for the same perfection.

When I arrived in Pittsburgh, I found someone who strove for that same standard of perfection, while also demonstrating a level of creativity in his work I had never witnessed before. That is why I chose to pattern myself after Cyril Wecht. As the two of us got to know one another, we found that we were quite similar, in spite of our very different backgrounds.

Spending time with Cyril and watching him do his thing was extremely enriching for me. Dr. Wecht is one of the best forensic pathologists in the world, and having the opportunity to learn from him in close quarters was nothing but divine providence. I was a blessed man. And a good student. I memorized everything he said to me, just like I had memorized the English alphabet and multiplication tables in early grade school.

One thing I learned from his personality was how not to speak your mind every time, especially in public. There are times you need to hold back, swallow your pride, walk away, and let things be, just like my mother advised me. There are times when the stronger and wiser man is the man who walks away from a fight. But sometimes you must stand your ground, no matter how many people are against you. That was Cyril Wecht. He showed me how to balance the two and how, when it was time to stand, to stand firm. In truth, he taught me the American swagger and how to use it.

For a forensic pathologist, one of the places where one must be most firm is the courtroom. When I was preparing for my first court case,

Dr. Wecht pulled me aside. "Bennet," he told me, "in the courtroom, you should never, ever change your mind or opinion on the witness stand. Your opinion is your opinion. It does not have to be right or wrong. It is your opinion, given as the expert you are. Look around you in the courtroom, and you will realize you are the only one present who best knows and understands forensic pathology. Hell, you're probably the smartest person in the room. Always bear that in mind."

I took his advice, as I always did. Whenever I testified, I expressed my opinion without wavering. However, just being decisive was not enough. Cyril explained the dynamics of a courtroom trial to me. I learned from him that there was a time to display showmanship and a time to be straightforward and serious.

• • • •

My fellowship in the Allegheny County medical examiner's office lasted twelve months. A few months before I had completed it, Dr. Rozin, the chief forensic pathologist, approached me with two questions. He asked if I would be willing to assist Dr. Wecht with his private consulting company, which conducted autopsies and provided medicolegal analysis and testimony in cases outside of Allegheny County. Immediately I said, "Yes." By this point, I had applied for and been accepted into my second fellowship program, this one in neuropathology at the nearby University of Pittsburgh Medical Center. Dr. Wecht had encouraged me to pursue the second fellowship.

Dr. Rozin then asked if I might be interested in helping out in the medical examiner's office on weekends and public holidays while I completed my second fellowship. "The quality of your work is excellent," he said. "Dr. Wecht and I would love to keep you and then hire you once you finish the second fellowship."

I was deeply humbled by the request. Now, completing a fellowship is not like taking night classes at the local community college. My duties within the neuropathology program were more than a full-time job.

While less than the eighty-plus hours per week that medical residents put in, a fellowship position still demands long hours. In spite of this, I jumped at the offer. "Yes, I would be honored to continue working with you," I said, even though my weekend work for the county, my private work for Dr. Wecht, and pursuing my second fellowship guaranteed I would not have a life outside of work for the next few years.

Over the course of the next year or so, Dr. Wecht entrusted me with more and more cases, especially those that needed to be done in a short time frame. In the beginning he had me do research for him. He then took my findings, studied them, made any corrections that were needed, and then presented them in his own voice. After I proved myself, he let me fly solo, taking on an entire case myself. Then, in the middle of 2001, he handed me a case where a man's life was literally on the line. I felt up to the challenge.

The case Dr. Wecht gave me involved a man named Thomas Kimbell. In 1998, Kimbell had been tried, convicted, and sentenced to death for a brutal, vicious quadruple murder. His first conviction was overturned on appeal. The appellate court ruled that a crucial witness's testimony should have been allowed in his trial. Even after winning his appeal in the summer of 2001, Kimbell remained in jail pending a retrial. All the evidence from his first trial still stood against him. If the defense went into the new trial with the same approach as the first, the outcome would most likely be the same. That is why they called the preeminent forensic pathologist in Pennsylvania for help. Dr. Wecht referred them to me.

Thomas Kimbell's lead attorney called me and set up a meeting with the entire defense team in one of the high-rise buildings in downtown Pittsburgh. In the meantime, he sent over the files on the case for me to examine. Even with all my other responsibilities, I had time to devote to the case because, in those days, I did not have a life outside of work and church. I was not married, although I had been engaged once. That relationship had not lasted, which gave me that much more time for work. I did not mind the long hours I put in. Between my two jobs, I made a very good living. I saved a great deal of my money, while also sending money to my parents and family in Nigeria. My father had long since retired, but government corruption in Nigeria cost him his pension. Sending my parents money each month was the least I could do to step in and help provide for them as they had once provided for me.

I dove into the Thomas Kimbell file in preparation for my meeting with his legal team. The case was chilling. On the afternoon of June 15, 1994, a thirty-four-year-old, 250-pound mother of two, Bonnie Dryfuse, was attacked in her New Castle, Pennsylvania, home. She fought desperately for her life. While she fought off her attacker, her seven-year-old daughter Jacquelyn and four-year-old daughter Heather ran off with their five-year-old cousin, Stephanie Herko, and hid in the bathroom. Bonnie's assailant stabbed her twenty-eight times, taking her life. The fatal wound came long before the assailant stopped stabbing her. I found many of her stab wounds came postmortem. After the killer finished with Bonnie, he stormed into the bathroom and stabbed Jacquelyn fourteen times, Heather sixteen times, and Stephanie six times. The latter was particularly savage, for one of the stab wounds cut through her entire neck. Just reading about the nightmare this woman and these innocent little girls endured made me sick. How could anyone commit such horrible acts?

The prosecution claimed that Thomas Kimbell committed these crimes during a burglary while intoxicated with cocaine. Kimbell was a slight man, standing five foot three inches tall and weighing only 120 pounds. Everyone in town knew him. He lived at home with his mother, was unemployed, and was known to use cocaine. On the day of the Dryfuse murders, he came into town in the morning, snorted some cocaine at 11:00 a.m., and claimed to have hitchhiked back home around lunchtime. Later that evening, he admitted to taking an old bicycle that did not belong to him. The next day, he checked himself into the Saint Francis Hospital of New Castle out of fear of losing control. The night before, he had hit his mother with an open hand and admitted to having problems with his temper over the previous few days. Police arrested him that night for the stolen bicycle. Witnesses reported seeing him in the vicinity of the Dryfuse house. Police questioned him about the killings, but Kimbell maintained his innocence. With no physical evidence linking him to the crime scene, police let him go.

Two and a half years later, he was arrested when witnesses came forward saying Kimbell had bragged about killing Bonnie and her little girls. Another two years passed before he was finally tried. Even though the prosecution still did not have any physical evidence linking him to the crime scene or the murders, Thomas Kimbell was convicted on four counts of first-degree murder and sentenced to death. His successful appeal of the verdict bought him a second chance to prove his innocence. That's when his attorneys contacted me.

As I dug through the autopsy reports, the witnesses' testimonies, and the evidence presented at the first trial, I discovered a photograph of the hands of an adult male among the hundreds of photographs connected to the case. The hands showed nail abrasions, along with other abrasions and contusions on his palms, hands, and fingers. Dried blood could be clearly seen beneath his fingernails. When I saw those photographs, I believed I was looking at the hands of the killer. I later learned these were not Thomas Kimbell's hands, but the hands of Thomas Dryfuse, Bonnie's husband. He was the first person on the scene. Curiously, Thomas Dryfuse did not immediately call 911 when he allegedly discovered the mutilated bodies of his wife, daughters, and niece. Instead he called his father, who came to the home before any police officers ever arrived.

Thomas Kimbell's hands had also been examined immediately after the murders. As luck would have it, by checking himself into a hospital the day after the murders, Kimbell was given a thorough physical examination. Doctors found no evidence of any abrasions or lacerations or any wounds or bruising of any kind, either on his hands or anywhere on his body. I found this very curious, because the crime-scene photos of Bonnie, along with the pattern of her wounds, showed she had fought back hard against her assailant. I also discovered within Thomas Kimbell's files a comment that indicated he suffered from a form of hemophilia, the bleeding disease. If this was indeed the case, his medical condition made him extra susceptible to massive bruising. If he had been in a fight, he'd be bruised and bloodied. But he was not. To me, this cast doubt on his guilt.

• • • •

My first meeting with Thomas Kimbell's legal team got off to a rocky start. The one attorney on the team who knew me was out of the office and running late. "Just go on to the office and introduce yourself," he told me over the phone.

Apparently he forgot to communicate a few details about me to his office staff. I arrived at the downtown Pittsburgh location and took the elevator up to the firm's floor. "My name is Dr. Bennet Omalu," I said to the receptionist. "I am here for a meeting."

The receptionist looked up at me with an antagonistic expression on her face. "What meeting? I'm not aware of any meeting," she said.

"I'm supposed to meet with a team of attorneys," I said.

"We don't have any meetings like that scheduled for today. Are you sure you're in the right place?"

"The lead attorney is running late. Perhaps I will just take a seat and wait for him to arrive," I said.

"Okay," she said in a dismissive tone.

I took a seat in the corner of the reception lobby and waited and waited and waited. From where I sat, I could see several white men in suits sitting in a conference room. They appeared to be waiting for someone. After several minutes, I decided to go into the conference room and introduce myself. "I'm Bennet," I said. "Dr. Omalu. I am here for a meeting."

One of the men looked up with a very disdainful look on his face. "No. There must be another meeting somewhere. Perhaps you should go see the receptionist," he said.

"I'm sorry," I said, embarrassed. Rather than speak to the receptionist again, I decided to sit back down in the reception area and wait for the attorney with whom I had spoken before. When I sat down, I glanced over to the receptionist's desk. She glared at me as if to say, *How dare you!*

Ten minutes later, one of the men from the conference room came out and asked the receptionist, "Has the doctor shown up yet?"

"No, sir," she said.

He glanced at his watch, obviously frustrated, and then looked around the empty reception lobby. He looked right past me. "Okay. Let me know when he gets here," he said as he headed back to the conference room.

Finally, the lead attorney came running out of the elevator, panting. He came right to me. "Bennet, I am so sorry I'm late," he said. He led me into the conference room and introduced me to the other lawyers. They were all waiting for a big doctor, one personally recommended by Dr. Cyril Wecht himself, the doctor who was going to rescue their client from death row. They never expected that doctor to look like me. Every face in the room turned bright red, all except mine. I felt sorry for them all. Rather than allow this slight to discourage me, it actually motivated me. Right then, I was determined to outperform their expectations, while also rewarding Dr. Wecht's faith in me.

My first meeting with Thomas Kimbell was even more awkward. Based on my hours of research, I had come to the conclusion that Kimbell was indeed innocent. If I believed him to be guilty, I would have told them that as well. To me, three compelling facts told me he could not have committed these crimes. First, the pattern of the murders did not fit the theory proposed by the prosecution. The multiple stab wounds fit the textbook definition of "overkill," especially the multiple stab and incised wounds that came postmortem. These wounds were excessive and unnecessary, especially if the motive was simply to kill, as would have been the case in a drug deal or burglary gone bad. The trauma pattern did not fit. It was consistent, however, with intrafamily homicide.

Second, the evidence showed that Bonnie Dryfuse had fought valiantly for her life. She sustained twelve severe defense wounds of her left upper extremity, including her palms and fingers. The fact that she did not have any defense wounds on her right side indicated that she had fought her assailant while demobilized, with her upper right extremity pressed on the wall or floor. It is medically or forensically unlikely that a five-foot-three, 120-pound man could pin a five-foot-four, 250-pound woman to the ground while also assaulting her with a knife.

Finally, if Kimbell had committed this crime and had somehow pinned Bonnie Dryfuse to the ground while savagely attacking her, his hands and body would have been covered with abrasions and contusions. This is especially true since his file stated that he had a form of hemophilia. If he did indeed have hemophilia, then his bruises would have been unmistakable. But his medical examination the day after the killings showed absolutely no evidence of bruising or abrasions. The lack of contusions and abrasions convinced me that it was impossible for him to have committed these crimes.

To prove my hypothesis scientifically, I had to draw blood from him and have it tested. That is why I went to see him in jail. His attorney had gained a judge's permission to draw his blood. One of his lead attorneys with whom I had been working went with me to the jail. The two of us went into a visiting area and waited for a guard to bring Thomas Kimbell in to us. As soon as Kimbell laid eyes on me, he turned to his lawyer and said very loudly, "I thought I asked you to find me a guy who knew what he was doing, the best in the field, and you bring me a black man?"

I ignored him, but his attorney was noticeably embarrassed. "Don't mind him," the attorney said to me. "Thomas is an idiot. That's how he ended up in this mess."

I drew the blood. Tests confirmed that he did indeed have a form of hemophilia. This was the final piece of the puzzle. I typed up my findings in a seventeen-page report and sent it to his legal team in late February 2002. Two months later, I appeared in court and testified on behalf of the defense. My appearance in court that day was re-created in the opening scene of the movie *Concussion*.

After my testimony, the jury found Thomas Kimbell not guilty and set him free. He came over to me in the courtroom, tears flowing from his eyes. He threw his arms around me (with the judge's permission), and whispered in my ear, "Thank you, thank you, thank you." It was a very different scene from the first time we met.

I left the courtroom that day very happy that I was a forensic pathologist. I do not feel like this every day. While writing this book, I accompanied sheriff's deputies into an overgrown field, trudging through mud and deep brush in my tailored suit and Johnston & Murphy Aristocraft shoes, until we came upon a partially decomposed body of a woman who had been allegedly murdered and dumped by a rural river in the delta. I drove home that day wondering if it was too late to change careers.

But on the day of the Thomas Kimbell verdict, I had no doubt that God had led me into this place. It is funny, looking back, to realize how I got here. All the life decisions I had made as an adult prior to coming to Pittsburgh were all based on what I did *not* want to do or be rather than on what I did. Yet God used those decisions to put me in the place where He wanted me. *His* will was done, not mine, and as a result, my life was changed.

Looking back at the Kimbell case, I do have one regret. We were able to show who did *not* kill Bonnie Dryfuse, her two daughters, and her niece, but the real killer was never found. Bonnie and her children and her niece did not receive justice. After Kimbell's acquittal, local police did not reopen their investigation. I believed the husband, Thomas Dryfuse, should have been investigated closely, but he was not. Neither he nor anyone else ever became a suspect. The real killer was never caught. Thomas Dryfuse died in a motor vehicle crash in 2011. Apparently he had become an alcoholic, drove while he was intoxicated, and collided head-on with another vehicle while driving in the wrong lane.

By the time I finished the Kimbell case, I did not have to fake who I was any longer. I had figured out who the best version of me was, whether I was in the autopsy room, courtroom, or in what little private life I had. The timing for my finding myself was truly an act of God. Now that I had found myself, God had a divine appointment awaiting me, one that I never could have kept if I were still in the wilderness searching for me.

Chapter Eleven

A Divine Appointment

On the afternoon of September 28, 2002, autopsy case A02–5214 was no different from any other case on which I had worked in the Allegheny County medical examiner's office. The body of a white male, fifty years old, lay on the same table near the exit where I'd performed my first autopsy in this office during my externship. Three years, more than a thousand autopsies,[1] and two completed fellowships later, I was a different doctor, a different pathologist, and a different man from the one who drove into Pittsburgh in October 1998. When I was handed autopsy case A02–5214, people within the Allegheny County medical examiner's office had already begun calling me Mini-Cyril. I took it as a compliment.

I had gone out to a club the night before autopsy case A02–5214. I found it to be the one way I could relax. When I went out, I'd nurse a drink for a couple of hours while standing next to a speaker, nodding my head to the music. Around 3:00 a.m., I went home and slept for a few hours before reporting for work. Since I was the youngest pathologist in the office—and the only single one—I pulled many of the weekend and holiday duties, except Christmas and Easter, which were covered by the one Muslim pathologist in our office.

My late night caught up with me the day of autopsy A02–5214, and I overslept. Hurrying to get dressed for work, I turned on the television and listened to the news headlines while dashing around my condo.

Everybody, it seemed, was talking about the same thing on all the morning news shows. A famous football player had just died. That didn't strike me as remarkable, since people die every day, a fact I knew all too well. However, something about the tone of the newscasts caught my attention. While reporters gushed about this man's life on the field, they vilified him for his post-football life. Apparently he had thrown all his money away and become bankrupt. He was living in his truck and on drugs, they said. "What a shame!" one said. "What a waste!" said another.

The contradiction in the way in which reporters described the man's life piqued my curiosity. How could a man go from a hero to a bum so quickly? I found their description of him very offensive. To me, his behavior indicated some sort of psychological disorder or illness. To speak ill of such a person struck me as the worst sort of insult. As a child of God, he deserved dignity and respect, especially now.

However, once I was out the door and on my way to my office I did not give the matter a great deal more thought. Like I said, I deal with death every day. On the drive from my condo to the office, I turned up the music in my car and prepared myself mentally for what I might face this day.

When I arrived at the office, I found news crews around the office. My technician, Mr. Robinson, ran up to me as soon as I walked into the lobby. "Hey, Bennet, Mike Webster is here."

"Why is there so much commotion around here?" I asked, ignoring his statement.

"I told you. Mike Webster is here."

"Who is Mike Webster?" I asked.

The lobby got quiet. I looked around. Everyone was staring at me. I had no idea why. Then it hit me. "Was he the guy on television this morning?" I said.

"Yes, now you're talking. Mike Webster was one of the greatest football players to ever play the game," Mr. Robinson replied.

"Okay," I said in a way that made it clear I had no idea who or what he was talking about. All I knew was that this man had some sort of problems that ended his life early. It was my job to discover why.

When I am assigned a patient on whom to perform an autopsy, I do my best not to assume anything going in. I once had a case where a teenage boy escaped from the county juvenile justice center, only to be found dead in the bushes, not far from where he climbed over the fence. The family cried out, alleging he had been killed by the police or someone else around the facility. When I examined the body, I found no evidence of blunt force trauma or any other signs of foul play. To me, it was clear that no one killed the boy, but that he had died of natural causes. But what were they? I requested some very sophisticated chemical analyses of his blood, which identified biochemical evidence of anaphylactic shock. That wasn't enough for me. Digging deeper, I found that the anaphylaxis was triggered by exposure to a certain type of pollen. I went back to his escape route and found that he had run through some bushes with plants that contained the particular type of pollen to which the boy was allergic. His exposure to the pollen triggered a severe hypersensitivity reaction, which precipitated the boy's sudden death. The case just confirmed that one cannot assume or settle for easy answers. The boy's family deserved the truth, as did the officers of the juvenile detention center who had been falsely accused. That's why I dug deeper. I always dig deeper. Doing so is not out of the ordinary for me. It is how I do my job.

Once I finally got to my office, I was handed a file on Mike Webster. In it I found his medical records and the preliminary report on his death from the hospital. His cause of death was listed as coronary atherosclerosis, or heart attack. Verifying that diagnosis is not a difficult process. However, based on all I heard on the television before going to the office, I suspected that more than heart disease was at play here.

After reading through Mike's file, I walked over to his body in the autopsy room. Looking at his face, I whispered to him, "Hi, Mike. I am Dr. Omalu. Bennet." I patted him on his shoulder. "Mike, I heard about your life and what people have said about you. I think they are wrong. You are not the loser people are making you out to be. I think something has hurt you. Something did this to you. But I need your help, Mike. I'm going to use all of my skills and all of my knowledge and all of my education to find out what has happened to you, but I cannot do this alone. Come with me. Walk with me. Guide me to the light of the truth."

The technician working with me didn't say a word. By this point, he was used to me doing things my "weird" way. I was different, and everyone knew it. I talked to Mike and my other patients many times in my heart and mind for a very simple reason: when I look into their faces, I do not see a dead body; I see myself. As I wrote about my very first autopsy, I know that could be me lying there. Someday it *will* be me. All of us will die. That is why I treat those who come into my autopsy room with the same dignity and respect that I hope is shown to me someday. Every human being is created in the image of God and therefore deserves respect and honor, even in death. The Golden Rule says to do to others as you would have them do to you. Death does not invalidate the Golden Rule. Mike Webster and I—we share a common humanity and a common spirit. That is why I spoke to him and asked for his help. Because of our shared humanity, I could not do a simple examination and call it a day. He might have died of a heart attack, but I knew something more had happened to him that ultimately took his life at the age of fifty. As a child of God, I owed it to him to keep looking until I found his answers.

• • • •

The Mike Webster autopsy was very routine. I knew his cause of death. It was already written out for me in black and white. "White male. Fifty years old. Suffered a massive heart attack." But the words in his file did not explain how a hero beloved and admired by the entire city of Pittsburgh had become a bankrupt, divorced, homeless man living in his truck. I suspected the answer to that mystery could be found in his brain.

The brain is such a complex and beautiful organ. If the body is a family, the brain is the spoiled youngest child. She is the most pampered organ, yet she finds a way to always get her way. I had recently completed a second fellowship at the University of Pittsburgh, this one in neuro-pathology. I pursued this fellowship because I wanted to understand this spoiled child that is the brain.

I ticked off all the boxes with Mike Webster to confirm the original diagnosis of his cause of death. Then I began searching for the causes of his mental illness. When I opened his skull, I expected to find a bruised, shriveled, and beaten-up brain. But everything appeared normal. There was no evidence of blunt force trauma that I could see with the naked eye. Disappointed not to find an easy explanation, I removed the brain and carried it over to my work station. I grabbed a knife and was just about to cut into the brain to look further when something stopped me. I dropped the knife in exasperation, doubt, and frustration. For a moment I just stood there, thinking. Then I turned to the second autopsy techni-cian in the room and said, "Would you please fix the brain for me?" To fix the brain, we have to submerge it in a chemical called formalin for at least two weeks. The brain is about 60 to 80 percent water, and in the natural state, it is as soft as Jell-O. To be able to study the brain micro-scopically, we first need to submerge it in formalin so that it hardens and can be processed.

I gave the order to fix Mike's brain, even though I knew the county would not cover the cost of the tests, since these tests went beyond the parameters of what was necessary to complete his autopsy and determine his cause of death. If I wanted to fix the brain and study it further, I was going to have to pay for it myself. This was not the first time I covered the expenses for extra tests, nor would it be the last.

"Why?" she asked in a tone that conveyed far more than her one-word answer. The two of us did not work well together. She often treated me with disrespect, regularly questioning my instructions and even raising her voice at me. Since I was the only physician in the office she treated like this, and since I was the only black doctor in the office, I wondered if race or the fact that I was born abroad might play a factor.

Her disrespectful tone was more than I wanted to hear at that moment. "Fix that brain!" I said firmly, somewhat putting her in her place. She did as I said, but I suspected she would report me to the office manager and to Dr. Wecht. However, if I had to choose between having a technician report me as insensitive or intolerant and failing to exhaust every path to find the cause of Mike Webster's demise, I gladly chose the former. I owed Mike that. I hope he would have done the same for me.

. . . .

Because I knew the technician would not only report me but also question my order to fix the brain, I called Dr. Wecht as soon as I finished the autopsy to explain my actions. He was very interested in my results. Like everyone else in the office, Dr. Wecht was a huge Pittsburgh Steelers fan. I remained very much on the outside looking in when it came to football. Even after living in Pittsburgh for three years, I knew no more about the game than I did the day I moved into the city. There were, I now know, football teams in Seattle and New York, but at the time, neither city matched Pittsburgh in its rabid love of the game or in its devotion to the home team in particular.

"So what did you find, Bennet?" Dr. Wecht asked on the phone.

"He died from a heart attack, just as the hospital said," I said.

"So that's it then?" he replied.

"I think there's more," I said.

"Oh," he said, surprised. "And what might that be?"

"I do not yet know, but I fixed his brain so I can study it further."

"And what do you think you might find?" His curiosity was piqued as well.

"I'm not sure, but something is not right. I saw the reports about him on the news this morning. From the description of his behavior and from his file, I suspected he'd suffered brain trauma. I expected his brain to appear abnormal. But it did not. Something did not match. Something just does not fit."

"Okay, Bennet. Good work. Let's talk about this Monday," Dr. Wecht replied.

I hung up the phone, returned to my desk, and wrote out the preliminary autopsy report. I filed it and went back into the autopsy room to do my work on one of the other bodies awaiting me. I walked over to the next person on whom I was to perform an autopsy and introduced myself. "Hello. I am Dr. Omalu. Bennet."

• • • •

Two weeks after Mike Webster's brain was fixed in formalin, I took it back over to my work station and resumed my examination of him. No one assisted me, because the office was not going to pay for unjustifiable testing. The cause of death was already determined, and all the proper documents had been signed. This was *my* quest for answers into what led to Mike Webster's death, not Allegheny County's quest.

I knew that Mike's heart gave out, but there was a very long pattern of behavior that defied explanation—behavior that ultimately led to the heart attack that took his life. The pattern actually started, but in a subtle manner, toward the end of his seventeen-year career in the National Football League. The symptoms progressed after his retirement. At first, he had trouble holding down a job. A series of poor business decisions and investments caused him to lose his house in foreclosure. He appeared both mentally and cognitively perturbed. Then he began to disappear for days at a time. He had memory losses, personality changes, disorientation, and spontaneous anger episodes.

Doctors prescribed medicines to help Mike. At different times, he took Prozac, Zoloft, or Paxil for depression; Ritalin or Dexedrine to keep him mentally alert; narcotic and nonnarcotic painkillers in various combinations (Tramadol, Propoxyphene, Hydrocodone) to ward off pain; Benzodiazepines to prevent panic attacks and anxiety; Selegiline to minimize movement disorders; and many others. But the drugs didn't help. It wasn't just the cognitive problems with which he had to deal; a lifetime of football left him in pain from the top of his head to the soles of his feet. Mentally, he became more and more lost. He sometimes forgot it was winter and went out in the freezing Pittsburgh weather without even a light jacket. He sank into paranoia and sleeplessness. At one point, he started using a Taser to shock himself to sleep.

As Mike sank deeper and deeper into mental illness, he visited some of the best neurologists and neurosurgeons in some of the best hospitals in the country. They ran all the latest, most thorough tests available, but no one could say exactly why Mike was the way he was. One of his doctors diagnosed him with post-concussion syndrome, among the many other diagnoses. That's the diagnosis that caught my attention, especially because Mike Webster had never officially sustained a diagnosed concussion. I also noted that Mike suffered from depression. That made him a kindred spirit to me. I did not know the cause of my depression. Perhaps I could give Mike the answers I never found for myself.

• • • •

Alone in the autopsy room, I cut into Mike's brain, not sure of what I might find. I took pictures with my own camera to document everything. To be honest, part of me just wanted to move on, but I had made a promise to Mike. I didn't want to go back on it.

To my surprise, everything in Mike Webster's brain looked completely normal. I became more confused. From everything I read about his long list of symptoms, he should have had visible signs of trauma or brain damage. But there were none. The more I looked, the more frustrated I became. In my subconscious, I just wanted out. Before I could, I needed to take one more step. I prepared brain sections that could be viewed under a microscope after they had been properly prepared. I took the sections to a lab at the hospital to a wonderful woman named Jonette Werley. She was the tissue histotechnologist who ran the brain tissue laboratory at the University of Pittsburgh Medical Center. We got to know one another during my neuropathology fellowship at the hospital.

Jonette took the sections of Mike Webster's brain and processed them for me. When she was finished, she placed them in my mailbox at the Presbyterian Hospital where I was an adjunct, or volunteer, clinical faculty member. And that's where the slides remained for the next several weeks. As I said at the beginning of the chapter, case A02–5214 did not stand out as anything unusual.

The extra steps I took to dig deeper into the real cause of Mike Webster's death were not unusual. I had done this with multiple cases. Mike's was not even the first brain on which I conducted such thorough analysis. Not long before Mike came into my autopsy suite, I conducted an autopsy on a woman named Florence. She lived in an abusive relationship with her husband. One night, he beat her up and pushed her down a flight of stairs. She suffered severe traumatic brain injury, with subdural hemorrhages. The fall did not take her life, not immediately at least. She lived in a vegetative state and passed four years later. I ordered the same types of tests on Florence's brain that I did on Mike's. In addition to the signs of the major trauma she suffered, I also found changes in her brain that resembled Alzheimer's disease, albeit with some slight differences. I paid for the analysis of Florence's brain out of my own pocket. I had to find answers for Florence, just as I did for Mike.

Looking back, if it hadn't been for Florence, I might never have had slides prepared of sections of Mike Webster's brain. And if I had never had slides prepared of Mike's brain, everything that follows in this book may have never happened. Florence prepared me for Mike—and I guess you could say Mike for me—but she was not the only one who played a role in bringing Mike and me together. I rarely watch television, especially in the morning, but I just happened to flip on the set the morning of Mike's death, which allowed me to hear the derogatory terms reporters used to describe his post-football life. When I heard he suffered from depression, my heart went out to him because I had suffered from it myself.

None of this would have meant anything if his body had come to the medical examiner's office during the week. Another doctor in the office would have handled his case, and I never would have become involved. But I was the doctor on duty, and I had a history of depression, and I had just completed a second fellowship in neuropathology, and I had just investigated the death of another patient who had suffered traumatic brain injury, which paved the way for me to conduct the same battery of tests on Mike. I was also the only forensic pathologist in the office who was a neuropathologist as well.

Autopsy case A02–5214 may not have initially jumped out at me as anything out of the ordinary, but looking back, I now realize this was truly a divine appointment. My life had led me to this moment and to this man. At the time, I had no idea the impact Iron Mike Webster would make on the rest of my life. If I had known, I probably would have walked away and dropped the case immediately. However, that is the thing about divine appointments. God reveals the details a little at a time as He takes us on His journey. It is up to us to trust Him, even when the road becomes treacherous.

Chapter Twelve

Prema

In July 2002, a couple of months before I met Mike Webster, one of the families in my church invited me to attend their daughter's wedding at our church's parish hall. I immediately accepted the invitation, even though I knew I would miss the ceremony and most of the reception. My church, St. Benedict the Moor, had become my second family. What little life I had outside of work I spent there. St. Benedict was actually the second church I attended after moving to Pittsburgh. The first, which was near my first apartment in a predominantly white part of Pittsburgh, did not exactly extend a warm welcome to me. One of the families in that church told me about St. Benedict, a predominately African–American church where many African immigrants also attended. From the moment I first walked in the door, I felt like I was home. Over time, I became more and more involved in the life of the church. I joined the choir, even though I cannot sing. When the sound system went out, I bought a new one for the church and even ran it during most services. It may be just my imagination, but I think the choir director preferred having me at the sound board rather than in the choir.

Because my church was family to me, I did not even consider declining the wedding invitation, even though I had to work that day. As soon as I finished my final report on my last autopsy of the day, I rushed home, took a quick shower, and dressed in my traditional Nigerian attire. I looked good, if I say so myself.

By the time I arrived at the parish hall, most of the other guests had already left. Only a few close friends and family were still hanging around. I went to the mother of the bride, whom I knew very well, and let her know I had arrived just as I had promised. She was very happy to see me. She fixed me a plate of food and then went to take care of the remaining guests. I was in a mood to chat, so I walked around the hall saying hi to everyone and cracking some jokes. As I walked around the parish hall, I noticed a group of about five young men and women sitting together in a corner, relaxing and chatting. They appeared to be a group of African students who had helped the mother of the bride serve food and drinks during the reception. Since most of the guests had already left, they had time to relax. They all appeared tired and were chilling out.

I headed over to the group for a very specific reason. In the middle of the group sat a long-haired young woman I had never seen before. I thought she was very cute, and this seemed the perfect time and place to introduce myself to her.

I walked over to the group of five in the corner. They were engaged in a conversation, but I ignored it. "Hi, I'm Dr. Bennet Omalu. It is good to meet you."

The five people in the group stopped talking and just sort of looked at one another. If I had paid any attention at all to them, I would have noticed the unhappy looks on their faces. I wasn't looking at anyone in the group except the one young woman with the long hair. I went straight to her and stretched out my hand. "It's really nice to meet you."

"How dare you!" she snapped back. Her accent appeared to be Kenyan.

"What?" I asked, surprised.

"Just who do you think you are that you can walk right over here and interrupt our conversation? Don't you see how rude that is?"

"Well, I . . ." I stammered.

She looked me over and the clothes I was wearing. "I bet you are Nigerian, aren't you? You Nigerians are all alike. You are all rude." She was really letting me have it.

"I'm very sorry," I said. I then tried to salvage the moment, and I smiled and said, "I just thought you were cute, so I wanted to meet you. What is your name?"

"My name! Why would I tell you my name? You have to be the tenth Nigerian man who has come up to me today and told me I was cute and asked me my name." After saying this, she sort of glared at me, letting me know the conversation was over.

I was dumbfounded and humiliated. I turned around silently and walked away in shame. As I walked away, I heard them making jokes and laughing at me. I avoided that corner for the rest of the night.

An hour or so later, I found the bride and groom, wished them well, and told them I needed to get home and get to sleep. It had been a very long day, and I had to work the next day. Before I could get out the door, the bride's mother called me. "Bennet, Bennet."

I turned and asked, "What can I do for you?"

"Can you drop off some of the workers who helped me tonight? They have put in a long day, and they do not have rides. I hate for them to have to go stand at a bus stop."

"Of course," I said, "I am glad to help. Just have them meet me at my car." I went outside and pulled my car closer to the door. There I sat for half an hour. Finally, the group of workers who needed rides came walking out. You can probably guess who they were. The people who needed a ride home were four of the five people in front of whom I had so embarrassed myself earlier. Three climbed into the backseat, while the girl with the long hair got in the front.

I did not make eye contact with her. Instead I asked the group, "Where do you need to go?" I drove each person to their address. One had forgotten her keys, so I drove back to the parish hall so she could retrieve them. Another had to pick up something from the pharmacy. I told her it would be no trouble to make an additional stop. After that, I had to stop by the grocery store on the way to the next-to-last address. I did not complain, nor did I say anything to the girl in the front seat.

Finally, I did have to speak to the girl. "What address do I need to take you to?" That was all I said. I didn't dare say anything after the tongue-lashing she'd given me earlier in the evening. She gave me an address. When we got to the house where she shared a room with a friend, she asked me, "Would you mind dropping me off at the laundry? It seemed everyone else needed to make another stop, and this would help me a lot."

"Of course I will take you," I said.

She disappeared into her house and emerged a few minutes later with a laundry bag. I drove her to the laundry, which was not far from her house. "Okay, this is it," I said. "Bye-bye."

Before she got out of the car, she smiled at me for the first time. "You are a very nice and patient man and not at all the jerk I thought you were," she said.

I smiled and said, "Thank you." I still did not know her name, nor did I dare ask. I just wanted to get home and go to sleep. This was not exactly the kind of night I wanted to remember.

The next day, I had forgotten about the girl and was consumed again by work. A very busy week went by filled with work and classes and everything else that packed my days to the maximum. The group of people I'd chauffeured after the wedding was the last thing on my mind when I arrived at church the following Sunday. That is, until I saw this same girl sitting on the other side of the sanctuary. Since she was at the wedding, I should have guessed she attended St. Benedict, but I had never noticed her before. In spite of the rough time she gave me at the wedding reception, I still thought she was cute.

After the service, I went to my pastor, Father Carmen D'Amico, and asked him about this woman. Father Carmen was more than my priest and pastor; he was like an older brother who profoundly impacted my life during my time in Pittsburgh. Before I became a part of St. Benedict, I had struggled in living out my faith. Father Carmen became a spiritual mentor to me. From him I learned how to live out a quiet and deep faith in my normal routines of life. The two of us got together on almost a daily basis after morning Mass. Over coffee, we talked about life and faith and everything else. More than what he said to me, he changed me by the way I watched him live out his faith. He inspired me to do more, to be more of a man of God.

Occasionally during our coffee talks, Father Carmen mentioned people within the congregation who needed help. Through his influence, I got involved in the evangelical ministry of the church, taking tapes of the services to our shut-ins who could not make it to church. I also delivered the Holy Eucharist to these same members. At the St. Benedict the Moor parish, I got to know many older African-American men and women who had lived through the darkest days of racism in our country. From them I learned how to respond to injustices in a Christlike manner. Later, when I experienced a different kind of opposition, I went back to the lessons I had learned from these dear people. They shaped how I respond to my critics even to this day.

I write all of this to let you know what kind of relationship I had with Father Carmen and the role he had in my life. I can honestly say that without his influence, I never would have survived the storm I encountered after I went public with what I discovered in Mike Webster. All of that was still in the future when I asked Father Carmen about this woman. "Who is she?" I asked.

"She is the woman about whom I spoke with you last week over coffee," he said. He had indeed mentioned a woman named Prema who had recently moved to Pittsburgh from Kenya by way of Michigan. Over coffee, he had told me she was attending a local community college to earn her nursing degree, but was having a difficult time. He asked me then if I might consider helping her, and I had told him I would. At the time, I had no idea that *this* was the woman he'd told me about.

"She's the one?" I said, surprised.

"Yes. That's Prema. Come, let me introduce you to her. I know you can help her. I feel the Spirit of God in you, Bennet. I know you will help as you have helped others in the parish."

"How can I help her?" I asked.

"Help her as a Christian brother helps his sister," he said.

To be completely honest, after the hard time she gave me when we first met, I was not completely sure trying to help her was such a good idea. However, I knew God spoke through my pastor. I followed him over toward her.

When Prema saw me approaching, she broke into a smile. That was a good sign. "Hi," she said.

"Hello," I replied.

"Good, the two of you know each other," Father Carmen said and walked away.

"Do you need a ride home?" I asked. "I can drive you."

"That would be nice," she said. We talked on the way home. Before we got to her house, I asked if she was hungry. That led to a detour for lunch. Reading all of this you might conclude that this was a romantic lunch. It was not. Romance was not on my mind, nor was it on hers. Yes, I thought she was cute, but after Father Carmen asked me to help her as a Christian brother, any thoughts of romance had to go away. He had entrusted her to me as an act of faith in my character. The last thing I would ever do was betray that trust. As a Christian brother, I decided to help her like I would help one of my sisters—Winny, Uche, or Mie-Mie.

• • • •

It quickly became clear what kind of help Prema needed. In addition to attending classes for her nursing degree, she also worked nights sorting mail for a large bank. After work, she rode the bus home, slept for two or three hours, got up, and went to class. I hated that she had to ride a bus late at night, so I volunteered to drive her when my job was less busy. One night, she called late at night, in tears. She'd been demoted to housekeeper after her supervisor made a pass at her and she rejected him.

That was the last straw for me. If Mie-Mie's boss had made a pass at her, I knew exactly what I would tell her. "I want you to quit your job and just concentrate on school," I told Prema.

"I have to work to live," she said.

"I have a very good job and make plenty of money," I told her. "I will support you until you get your degree."

The mention of a degree was a sore point for both of us. Prema already had a degree from a college in Kenya. However, many places in the United States did not recognize her degree or equate it to a nursing degree obtained from a school in the United States. That's why she had gone back to school.

"We can find you an apartment closer to the school. Do not worry. I will cover the expenses until you graduate and get on your own feet," I said. Prema hesitated. "Do not feel bad because you have a need. Need is not bad. Need is need. As part of the one body of Christ, this is how we are to help one another. Please, let me do this for you."

There is an old African saying that goes, "Your fellow human being is the God you see and the God you know." First John 3:17–18 says very much the same thing: "If someone who has worldly means sees a brother in need and refuses him compassion, how can the love of God remain in him? Children, let us love not in word or speech but in deed and truth." When we have a need, God does not come down from heaven to meet that need Himself. Instead, He sends our fellow human beings to be His angels of mercy, grace, peace, and love. He has sent so many angels into my life at just the right moment. I felt privileged to be the angel in return.

I helped Prema find a place to live in a better part of town, along with paying her rent and tuition and giving her a weekly living allowance of a couple hundred dollars. For me, this was a way of repaying the kindness my sisters and their husbands and my extended family showed to me when they helped cover my expenses in coming to America. This was not about love. I didn't even know what love was.

There was, however, a day I believe I fell in love with Prema without even knowing it. One afternoon I picked her up to help her run some errands when she turned to me and asked, "Would you take me to the Western Union office so I can wire some money to my mother back in Kenya?"

"Okay," I answered in a puzzled tone. I knew Prema barely had enough money to make it week to week.

She sensed my wonderment and answered the question I did not dare ask. "My father left my mother unannounced one day and married a younger woman. Since then, my mother was on her own with us and raised me, my sister, and our two brothers. I send her money every month, if you must know."

"You did not need to tell me all of this, but I am grateful you did," I said, once again humbled by this woman. I never quite looked at her the same way again, for now I had seen her heart. She cared more for others than she did for herself—to such a degree that she sacrificed for them. This was a woman who was not afraid to love. When I first saw her, I thought she was cute, but now I saw a beauty I cannot describe. I took her to Western Union, where she wired money to her mom. After that, I stepped up my own care for her. If I noticed she needed something, I acted.

• • • •

About a year after first meeting Prema, we entered into a romantic relationship. I should have been thinking about marriage from the start. After all, I was in my mid-thirties when we started dating. Dr. Wecht had already been after me to get a life outside of work. I spent a lot of time with his family. Over and over, he told me, "Bennet, you need to get married and start a family of your own."

Dr. Wecht wasn't the only person telling me I needed to get married. On New Year's Day 2005, I called my family in Nigeria. Each one asked me about my plans for the new year. Then all of them, from my mother and my father down to my sisters and brothers, said, "You should think of getting married." I got very frustrated. Finally, I turned to Prema, who was with me in my condo, and blurted out, "Are you ready to get married? Will you marry me?"

She laughed at me. "If you want to marry me, I will marry you," she replied.

I grinned. "Yes, let us get married. We will fall in love as we live together in our old age." At the time, I did not know or understand what love is. I do now. Asking Prema to marry me is the best decision I have made in my life. She is a gift from God.

In December 2005, three years after we first met, Prema and I flew to Enugu, Nigeria, where we were married with our families in attendance. I stood in amazement as she walked down the aisle with her younger brother, Tom, to me standing at the altar next to Father Carmen D'Amico, who officiated our wedding. Prema looked like the angel that she is. With each step she took, I prayed in my heart that the good Lord would give me the strength, courage, and wisdom to love and cherish her, stand by her, uplift her, and support her to become the woman she was born to be, to be the wind beneath her wings that will make her soar as high as she can to be herself, fulfill her dreams and aspirations, and reach for the heavens in our lives together. I vowed to God and myself that I would always be there for her and remain an angel of God to her, until death do us part. As my father advised me, I chose that day to love her and share my life with her for the rest of my life. Every day I reaffirm that decision in my heart.

Prema is such an important part of this story, and not just because she became my wife. The wedding reception where we first met occurred a couple months before I met Mike Webster. As I began to research Mike's condition and as that research expanded beyond what I ever imagined possible, Prema stood beside me. I soon found myself up against those who tried to discount my research from the start, but she was an opposite voice, encouraging me to believe in myself and to trust my research. Without her, the story ends here. Thankfully, our story—together—is still being written to this day.

Chapter Thirteen

A Game-Changing Diagnosis

One Friday afternoon in 2003, several months after Mike Webster's autopsy, I finally got around to taking a look at the slides of his brain. I was tired from a long day of work, where I was so busy I didn't even have time to eat lunch. The clock read 5:00 when I got back to my cubicle of an office. I was munching on a red apple when I glanced up and noticed a box of slides on one of my shelves. About a month earlier, I'd pulled the slides out of my box at the hospital, not because I planned on working on them right away, but because my box was full. That day, I tossed them on my shelf and told myself I would get around to them eventually. Eventually came this day—this late Friday afternoon when my stomach was empty and my body was tired, but I needed to stick around the office to get some work done.

I pulled the set of slides off the shelf, took one out, and placed it on the tray of my office microscope. This microscope, like everything else in my cubicle office, was anything but state of the art. Honestly, it should have been in a high school classroom, not in a medical examiner's office, but it was what I had been given to work with. The computer I used was just as outdated, but I made do with what I had. Such is the nature of working in a government office where the manager does not like you and you are at the bottom of the seniority scale.

Even with the inferior quality of my office microscope, it was clear something was not right with the cells on these slides. Under normal circumstances, brain cells are a work of art under a microscope. A healthy brain cell resembles a bright, full moon rising above the horizon on a cool, clear October night. Its beauty is nearly indescribable.

I did not see a thing of beauty on the first slide I examined. In fact, I pulled the box of slides back down from the shelf and double-checked to make sure I had the right brain. Yes, the box of slides was labeled Case A02–5214, Mike Webster.

These slides did not appear like they should belong to a fifty-year-old man. Each slide contained numerous brain cells, yet many had died and disappeared, and many appeared like ghost cells. A large number of the remaining cells appeared shriveled, as if in the midst of the throes of death. I observed spaces—spongiosis—in the substance of the brain, with shriveled brain skeleton and skeins of brain scars, like a partially demolished building stripped of its windows and its aesthetics gone, leaving behind just the main frames, pillars, and broken-down walls.

In the midst of this broken-down building, I observed ugly threads and fibrils of brownish proteins inside and outside the brain cells. I recognized them as tau proteins. Tau protein in a healthy brain is part of the skeleton of the brain cells and fibers. They provide both support and transport nutrients up and down the brain cells and fiber. When a person sustains a blow to the head and sustains either a concussion or subconcussion, the skeleton of the cells and fibers fracture. Because the brain cannot heal like the skeleton of the body, the proteins begin to form abnormal "strangle proteins" that eventually kill the brain cells. For most people, the loss of a few brain cells is not a problem, since we have billions. However, when the strangle proteins spread throughout the brain, the damage results in symptoms like Mike Webster demonstrated. The patterns and distributions of these abnormal proteins I found in his brain were also surprising because they looked different from the patterns and distributions we see in patients suffering from other types of dementia, including Alzheimer's disease. I did not expect to see any of these in the brain of a fifty-year-old former athlete. With this first look through the microscope, I could not yet know the extent of the damage, nor did I see everything I just described during this initial observation. These discoveries unfolded over the course of months.

After my initial observation, I took the slides home to study them with my own equipment, which was significantly better than the microscope in my cubicle. Believe it or not, I did not immediately jump on the slides. When I returned home late that Friday night, I went out to relax. (Prema and I had not yet started dating.) By the time I got home, I had more pressing matters than slides connected to a six-month-old autopsy case. I placed the slides on top of my desk and basically forgot about them.

Looking back, I realize I didn't just forget about the slides. I knew they were there, but I was hesitant to study them further. Here is why: A short time after I moved to Pittsburgh, one of the autopsy technicians who had worked in the medical examiner's office invited me to a get-together at his home on a Sunday afternoon. Joe is a big, gregarious Italian guy who loves to cook and entertain. I gladly accepted his invitation, although I got there a little late on the day of the party. When I walked in, Joe handed me a beer and began introducing me to the thirty or so people who were there. Some I knew from work. It was a nice mix of people, with everyone from neurosurgeons to blue-collar types. Everyone seemed to be enjoying themselves, while the wonderful smell of the food was nearly intoxicating. I was glad to be there.

I found a place to sit. The television was on, and most of the other guests were glued to it. I glanced over, wondering if some news story had broken. Instead I saw a game was on. Sports wasn't much of an interest of mine at the time. When I was a boy in Nigeria, I used to keep up with soccer, but only casually. I also ran track in my early teenage years, but that was the extent of my personal involvement in sports. Nothing changed after I moved to the States. I worked so many hours during my residency and fellowships that there wasn't much time left over for such pursuits.

The people at the party, however, grew more and more passionate about the game on the television. They yelled and screamed and moaned and cheered with every play. They weren't just *watching* the game. As I settled into my seat and started watching the people around me, I noticed an intense debate going on in the room. I listened closely, but the subject made no sense to me. This argument was also odd because most of the people in the room agreed with one another, but that only seemed to make them get louder and more animated in their discussion. It seemed that they were all quite upset with the quarterback of the Pittsburgh Steelers. I had no idea what a quarterback was, and my only exposure to the Pittsburgh Steelers was seeing the name on shirts, hats, and jackets everywhere I went in the city. At least half of the people in the room on this day had on some sort of Steelers attire.

The game on television, it seemed, was not going well, which only made the debate about the quarterback grow even more intense. From what I could gather, the Steelers quarterback was a young African-American man, and most in the room doubted he was ever going to be any good. The majority seemed to think he needed to be replaced. As the game wore on, the feeling that he should be replaced grew stronger and louder. Of course, the alcohol being consumed by the party guests may have also had something to do with that sentiment. The debate continued when the food was served—and all the way through to the end of the game.

That's when I left. I thanked Joe for having me over and told him I had a wonderful time. However, as I left his house, I had this feeling that I had just witnessed some sort of an odd religious sect or a cult, like an anthropologist who stumbles upon a ritual ceremony in a clearing in the middle of a rain forest under a starry sky. The emotions and passion in the room surpassed those I observed at any ordinary church service. As Cyril Wecht told me later, when I was neck-deep in my fight with the National Football League, football truly owns a day of the week— the same day the church used to own. God no longer has any claim to Sundays, at least not in Pittsburgh, between Labor Day and Valentine's Day. Sundays belong to football.

Why would that matter to a scientist in search of truth? Deep in my spirit, I had a feeling that if I pulled out those slides and dug deeper into

Mike Webster's brain, whatever I might discover was going to put me in direct conflict with the passion for football that consumes Pittsburgh and most of America. Conflict never comes at a good time, and this was the worst possible time for me to put myself at odds with my colleagues and my community. My career as a pathologist was really just getting started. I had completed a second fellowship in neuropathology less than one year earlier and was already thinking of working toward a master's degree in public health. Dr. Wecht had a law degree and had encouraged me to think about going to law school. Law school would be a giant step for my career, a step that would take me even closer to fully realizing the American Dream that attracted me to this wonderful country in the first place.

That is why I let the Mike Webster slides collect dust on my desk. If I pulled them out and examined them thoroughly, the future about which I dreamed, the future that was well within my grasp, might well be at risk. Knowing that, I did not know if I had the courage to go through with what I knew I needed to do.

And yet I had made a promise to Mike Webster, and his spirit would not let me forget it.

• • • •

One evening, I came home late and happened to look over at my desk. There sat the box of slides. I summoned the courage to take another look. The ghost cells and strangling tau proteins popped out at me. *Why are they there, and how widespread are they?* I wondered. Over the next few months, I either stayed up late at night or got up early each morning and went through slide after slide, observing damaged cell after damaged cell. I stared at those cells so many times that I could close my eyes and still see them and every detail about them. My mind became consumed with understanding what I was observing. Sometimes I woke up in the middle of the night and went straight to my microscope. The search for the truth became my life.

I had more slides prepared from other parts of Mike's brain. All showed the same fibrils and threads of tau proteins branching out like a sickly tree, entangling and essentially strangling the brain cells. Interestingly, as I examined more slides, I began to notice another type of abnormal protein that should not have been there—the diffuse amyloid protein plaques that were scattered in different regions of his brain and doing the same thing tau proteins did, creating a toxic environment for brain cells. I got totally confused. I did not understand or know what I was looking at. My puzzlement only became agitated. I could not rest until I found the answer.

As I wrote earlier, a healthy brain cell is a thing of beauty, but that beauty had been lost in Mike Webster. The tau and amyloid proteins left many of the remaining brain cells little more than mummified remains of their former selves. It wasn't just the presence of these proteins that I found alarming, but how uniquely distributed they were in the brain. I had not watched much football, but I knew that very large men collide headfirst multiple times throughout a game. Even though they wear helmets, their brains are not protected. A helmet keeps someone from lacerating their scalp, breaking their skull open, or suffering some type of bleeding inside the skull. It does not cushion the brain as it impacts the inside of the skull in a headfirst collision of bodies. Nothing can protect the brain in such an impact.

The images I observed under my microscope stirred my curiosity. I believe America is the most intelligent country in the world, so surely some American must have already described what I was seeing in great detail. After all, football is the most popular sport in America, and the NFL is its most popular and richest league. I started searching all the published literature I could find regarding brain trauma and dementia. For months, I went to the medical library at the University of Pittsburgh and checked out one medical journal after another. In those days, most journals did not have electronic versions. I read the physical copies. Many times the library did not have the journal I needed. I then turned in an order form for the paper I needed, and someone photocopied the pages I requested and brought them to the circulation desk.

One day, I received a phone call from one of the librarians. "Are you Bennet Omalu?" he asked.

"Yes."

"Then you are a real person?"

I laughed. "I believe so," I said.

"May I ask you a question?" He sounded rather hesitant.

"Of course."

"You have ordered a very large number of journals and research papers through the library. May I ask why?"

"I am a neuropathologist working in the Allegheny County coroner's office. I am currently doing research for one of the cases on which I am working," I said.

The librarian let out a little sigh. "Thank you. I am sorry I had to call and ask, but with the unusual volume of requests you have turned in, we needed to verify that you were, in fact, a real person with a genuine need for these papers."

"I can assure you I am real. I very much appreciate all of your staff at the library. You have all been invaluable to my research," I said. The librarian did not call back, even though I continued ordering a large number of papers from the medical library.

The more I searched for answers, the more amazed I became that no one had ever reported the phenomenon I had observed in Mike Webster. The tau tangles and amyloid plaques resembled Alzheimer's disease but did not look exactly like Alzheimer's disease. As I have already written, Mike was far too young to have Alzheimer's disease. Also, the patterns, while similar, were distinct from each other. I also researched dementia pugilistica, or punch-drunk syndrome, in boxers. The discovery of that syndrome proved to be quite controversial when papers describing it were first published in the late 1800s and early 1900s. Back then, boxing was one of the most popular sports in America, but the discovery of dementia pugilistica threatened its popularity. However, I knew I had found something different, because the punch-drunk brain frequently shows some physical damage that can be observed with the naked eye.

Mike's brain did not. Whatever I had observed in Mike Webster's brain was unique.

All we know and have known about blunt force trauma to the head makes it clear that single, episodic, and repetitive blows to the head have the potential to cause permanent brain damage. It makes no difference whether the blows come in sports venues or outside of them. Boxing, obviously, involves blows to the head. Yet, from what I could find, nothing had been reported in any other contact sport regarding brain disease—not in football or rugby or ice hockey or martial arts. I found this hard to believe. How could I, an immigrant doctor working in a coroner's office in the middle of Pennsylvania, be the first to discover what appeared to be a new disease? This just did not seem possible. Yet all of my research led me to one conclusion: this was indeed something new—a new disease that attacks the brain.

Now I had to answer a second question: What caused it? I could not say just football had done this to Mike Webster. As a scientist, I had to have proof to establish such a connection. Therefore, I began to study the game and what happens physically to those who play it.

When we look at football from a scientific posture, we find a game where large amounts of kinetic energy are transferred to the bodies of players in what is called biomechanical loading. When two players collide, or when one player collides with the ground, this is called *impact* biomechanical loading. The brain is most vulnerable during this kind of impact, because the brain itself essentially floats inside the skull. When the body abruptly stops, the brain continues to move until it slams against the inside of the skull. When the Jell-O–like soft brain that is 60 to 80 percent water hits against the inside of the skull, the microscopic support structures of the brain fracture slightly. Even more damaging is a hit that is off-center, which causes the brain to experience rotational acceleration where the brain essentially spins within the skull, resulting in sheering damage.

Now, this sort of impact can happen to anyone, and it does. When you get up in the middle of the night and bang your head against the wall while trying to find the bathroom, you have experienced an impact biomechanical loading. That does not lead to strangling tau proteins across your brain, nor does it normally lead to memory loss, violent mood changes, and the other behavior changes exhibited in Mike Webster, changes that began even before his football career ended.

Here's what made Mike Webster's experience unique, and what led me to believe that football was at the root of this new disease: a football player can undergo impacts at a velocity between 17 and 25 miles per hour. This results in rapid changes in head and brain velocity that can reach 20.1 miles per hour. The brain then experiences a peak acceleration–deceleration that can reach 138 gravitation (g) force and last up to 15 milliseconds. That's like getting hit in the head by a 10-pound cannonball traveling 30 miles per hour.[1] Another way to think of it is like being in a car wreck. That's what Mike Webster called it. When asked if he had ever been in a car wreck, he said, "Oh, probably about 25,000 times or so."[2]

One of the myths I found perpetuated as I started researching Mike Webster's case was that such blows to the head, even those that resulted in a concussion, were thought to be minor injuries. Concussions themselves are officially referred to as *mild* traumatic brain injury. Think about that for a moment. How can anything be both mild and traumatic? Concussions were considered so trivial in football that throughout most of its history, unless a player was knocked out cold, both the player and the team ignored it. Some physicians have proposed that there are three grades of concussion. Symptoms of a grade one concussion include seeing stars after a blow to the head. A retired NFL tight end interviewed for this book said he saw stars in practice or in games at least once a week. Not surprisingly, he is now dealing with memory loss, even though he is only in his mid-thirties. Other players report seeing stars multiple times in a single game, sometimes more than once on a single play.

The question I then had to answer was whether or not these repeated blows to the head were responsible for the damage I found within Mike Webster's brain. My research into brain disease took me all the way back to the time of Hippocrates four hundred years before the birth of Christ. It is a well-established fact that exposure to all types of blunt force trauma to the head damages the brain and leaves permanent sequelae, or pathological condition resulting from the injury. That is exactly what this appeared to be—a lasting pathological condition that resulted from repeated blows to the head. I explored other possible causes for what I had observed, including drug use, steroids, and genetic factors. None could explain the tau fibrils running through the brain, choking out brain cells. Blunt force trauma was the only plausible explanation based upon the research I conducted. The damage in Mike's brain was not a side effect of any of the medications he had taken. It was not the result of any kind of alcohol or drug use, including anabolic steroids. Blunt force trauma, both concussive and subconcussive, was the culprit.

This, then, was where I found myself. I believed I had discovered a new brain disease that was caused by repeated blunt force trauma to the head—trauma related to that experienced while playing the game of football. This disease was, I believe, responsible for Mike Webster's erratic behavior, as well as the depression, memory loss, mood swings, poor decision making, and the other odd characteristics that marked his life after football. Right away, I knew this was going to be a game changer for American football. Naively, I thought the world of football would welcome my findings with open arms.

• • • •

One day while driving home from work, stuck in traffic, I wondered what I should do next. I had become so engrossed in my research that I became somewhat overwhelmed by what I was doing and experiencing. Two types of fear came over me: the fear that I was wrong or delusional, and the fear of the impact my discovery was going to have. I had to show my research to another pathologist to confirm what I had seen or to have him show me why I was wrong. Bringing in another pathologist is the standard of practice set by the College of American Pathologists.

It dictates that when a pathologist sees an unusual case, he or she should show it to a second pathologist to confirm his or her findings. I knew exactly to whom I needed to go.

When I reached my home, I called one of my neuropathology professors, Dr. Ronald Hamilton, at the University of Pittsburgh. During my fellowship in neuropathology, Dr. Hamilton had trained me in the art and science of diagnosing neurodegenerative diseases of the brain and dementias. He had a great impact on my life, not only as a pathologist, but also as a human being and the way in which I perceive those with lifestyles different from my own. For this I am eternally grateful to him.

There is a scene in the movie *Concussion* that re-creates the moment Dr. Hamilton first observed the slides of Mike Webster's brain. The movie's depiction is very accurate. Dr. Hamilton knew immediately the possible repercussions of this discovery. "We need to show this to Dr. DeKosky," he said. Dr. Steven DeKosky was the head of the department of neurology at the University of Pittsburgh and one of the country's leading experts on Alzheimer's disease. When Dr. Hamilton mentioned Dr. DeKosky's name, my first thought was, *I don't think he will want to see me.* The two of us had only interacted slightly during my neuropathology fellowship. Basically, the few times I had run into him in the hospital, he had completely ignored me. After all, I was just a fellow, and he was the head of the department.

I thought I would be given perhaps five minutes maximum of Dr. DeKosky's time. Instead, the two of us spent at least two hours discussing this case, football, and life in general. Before I left that meeting, it was clear that I needed to publish my findings. Dr. DeKosky asked if he could be a coauthor—a suggestion I gladly welcomed.

When I left Dr. DeKosky's office, I was more excited than I had ever been. Not only had I discovered a seminal case with possible wideranging repercussions, but one of the leading scientists in the country had agreed to coauthor my research with me, as did Drs. Hamilton and Wecht. In that moment, I really thought this paper had the potential to do a great deal of good for very many people. Not only did I believe I had restored Mike Webster's humanity, but I also thought this research could help the many others I suspected were suffering silently with the same disease. This research, this paper I was to pen, was for them, not for me. This was not about building a name for Bennet Omalu, but about raising awareness of the danger of America's game and, as a result, protecting future players from the fate that befell Mike Webster.

How could I have been so naive?

Chapter Fourteen

Nearly Over before It Begins

My efforts to go public with what I had discovered in Mike Webster's brain nearly did not happen. The biggest culprit was not the National Football League, nor was it the antiquated system in which medical research is conducted in the United States today. Neither of those made my work any easier, but they did not stop me in my tracks and threaten to end all of my work before it really even started. No, that distinction falls to a primitive, inhuman, and inhumane system with which the vast majority of Americans will never interact. My life's work was nearly stopped completely by the United States immigration system and its set of arcane rules.

I came to the United States at the age of twenty-six on a visiting scholar visa. There are numerous categories of visas, and this was the one I was granted to come to America for the program at the University of Washington to which I had been accepted. After my year in Washington, I renewed my visa with the same category when I entered residency training and later when I started my first fellowship in Pittsburgh. However, as strange as it may sound, my visa required me to leave the country once a year and have my visa renewed there. I could not go to an immigration office in New York or Pittsburgh. Instead I had to travel to Canada or Mexico or even go back home to Nigeria and go through the renewal process at an American embassy. Renewing my visa required me to wade into the gargantuan bureaucracy of filling out confusing forms and answering questions in an interview with an official of varying temperament. Some of the interviewers were quite pleasant. Others spoke down to me and acted like I was a convicted felon applying for parole rather than a legal immigrant and future citizen of the United States of America. I soon learned I needed to have an immigration attorney accompany me to guide me through the process and deal with unexpected surprises. All in all, remaining a legal immigrant to the United States was very expensive and time-consuming.

In the spring of 2005, in the middle of revising and completing my academic paper on the Mike Webster case, I had to drop everything and take off for a week to go to Mexico for the annual visa renewal process. Up until 2005, I normally went to Toronto or Montreal. They were closer, and Canadians speak English. However, some United States embassies in Canada instituted new rules and changes that made it very difficult for my immigration attorney to accompany me. I'd been through this process enough times to know I needed my lawyer with me. My attorney recommended we go to Nogales, Mexico, instead of to Canada. Looking back, it was a wise choice.

One Monday morning, I flew from Pittsburgh to Tucson, along with about a half dozen to a dozen other people in the same boat as me. That night, we stayed in a nice resort on the outskirts of Tucson and then drove down to Nogales early the next morning. If everything went according to plan, we would return to Arizona that night. Nogales is a border town, with a town in Arizona and one in Mexico of the same name.

The drive down Interstate 19 took us through desert mountains and hills covered with majestic cactuses. The dry desert landscape could not have been more different from the deep greens of western Pennsylvania. Yet I found it to be beautiful, just one more expression of the incredible diversity of America. After perhaps an hour's drive, we arrived in Nogales, Arizona. Above the city sat huge, beautiful, multimillion-dollar homes on hills looking down on the valley below. The undulating hills stretched on before us, but the further south we went, the looks of them drastically changed. I could not see a visible line drawn in the sand, but as we crossed the Mexican border, the huge estates were replaced with shanties and abject poverty. It was as though I had crossed over into a completely different world.

The distinction between the wealth of America and poverty of Mexico could not have been more glaring. My mind went back to the questions I used to ask when I lived in Nigeria, where a sharp distinction was drawn between different parts of the country. Looking around Nogales, I was right back there again. The images made me angry, but I did not have time to dwell on it, because I had business that had to be done.

My attorney helped me and the rest of the group through the border crossing. From there, we headed straight for the American Embassy. All of us already had visa interviews scheduled. I had filled out all of the necessary forms and had my attorney double-check them to make sure everything was in order. The interview itself would take less than a half hour. However, there was always a delay between the interview and the actual visa stamp being issued. That meant we would all go out to lunch, pick up our visas in the afternoon, and be back in Tucson in time for dinner that night.

A ridiculously long line stretched out from the embassy gate. If we had to wait in that line, we might not get back to Tucson for a day or two. Thankfully, because we had appointments, our attorney was able to speed us through the line and into the waiting area within the embassy walls. The difference between the scenery inside and outside the embassy gates was also dramatic. The moment you walked into the embassy, everything had the look and feel of the United States. If I did not know I was in Mexico, I might well have believed I was back in Pittsburgh, albeit a hotter and dryer version.

I took a seat in the waiting area and waited my turn. As was now my habit, I wore a tailored suit and tie and designer shoes. My wardrobe reflected the influence of Cyril Wecht. He pulled me aside one day and told me that if I wanted people to take me seriously, I needed to dress like a successful medical professional. Down in Nogales, I was one of the few dressed so formally. All sorts of people filled the waiting area.

Above the room were photographs of then president George W. Bush and the secretary of state Colin Powell. One by one, members of my group had their numbers called and made their way to the counter for their interviews. I waited with eyes closed, trying to relax.

At long last, I heard someone call my number. I gathered all my papers and went to the counter where the interview was to take place. The word *interview* may conjure up an image of sitting down with an immigration official, perhaps across from a desk, but that is not the case. The visa interview is conducted at what most closely resembles a very secure bank lobby or prison visiting area. Just like in Lagos, Nigeria, a thick pane of glass separated me from a lovely, thirtysomething-year-old Hispanic woman. I spoke to her through a small speaker in the glass.

"May I please have your papers?" she said with a very kind tone. I passed them to her through a slot at the bottom of the glass. As she thumbed through them, she asked me a handful of questions. I answered each as best I could. With each answer, she checked off a box on a document I could not see. Once or twice, my attorney stepped in to help me answer the questions she asked. After a couple of minutes, she looked up from the pile of papers, smiled, and said, "Everything seems okay. Please have a seat in the waiting area, and I will be back with you in a couple of minutes." My attorney explained that she had to do a security check before she could approve my visa. "It's just a formality," he said. "There shouldn't be any problem, since you've already been in the country for many years now."

I sat down with the rest of my group. Everyone else had already been approved and were anxious to get to lunch. What should have been at the most a five-minute wait turned into ten minutes, then fifteen, then twenty. Members of my group fidgeted. None of us knew one another outside of this little trip to Mexico. The feeling in the group seemed to be, *Why is this guy making us wait?* Finally they all went outside to wait.

Thirty minutes after my interview, the woman who had interviewed me asked me to return to her window. My attorney whispered to me on the way up, "This is unusual."

As soon as I got to the window, the woman called me by my first name. Her tone had changed from sunny to concerned. "Bennet, there's a problem."

My heart sank.

"What is it?" my attorney asked.

"Bennet's name is listed on the security alert list."

"The what?" I asked.

"The security alert list. These are people who are wanted or who are suspected to be a risk to the United States. After 9/11 we have cracked down on any potential threats. For some reason, your name is now on that list," she explained.

I was dumbfounded. "How is that possible?" I asked. "Someone else must be using my name. I am a doctor. I work for the Allegheny County medical examiner's office in Pittsburgh. How could I possibly be on a security alert list?"

"I thought about that, and so I double-checked the information. I confirmed that indeed the person on the list is Bennet Omalu from Nigeria with your same birthday. It is you," she said.

I glanced over at my attorney. The look on his face told me this was serious trouble. "So what does this mean?" I asked.

"It means you will not be allowed to return to the United States," she said.

Those words would have been devastating enough if I were just a visitor to the United States, but my life was there. My closest friends were in the U.S., my fiancée, my life's work, to say nothing of everything I owned in this world. Now all of it was about to be stripped away from me. "What can I do?" I asked.

"It seems your name was added to the list by the American Embassy in Nigeria where your original visa had been issued. Because they added it to the list, they have to remove it. I'll contact them and see if I can discover what's going on over there." She smiled to try and reassure me, but it did not help.

My attorney requested to speak with the consul to discuss my case and receive further clarification. I went back to the waiting area. A short time later, my attorney came back and motioned for me to follow him outside. There we found the rest of our group, hungry and restless. They picked up very quickly on what was going on. My attorney pulled me aside and said, "Bennet, I have to take the rest of the group back to Tucson. Unfortunately, you will have to stay here. The lovely woman in the embassy has initiated the process of removing your name from the list, but it's going to take some time."

"How much time?" I asked. I was not equipped to stay in Mexico for even one night. My luggage was back in Tucson waiting for me. I didn't even have a toothbrush with me.

"It may take several hours, or it may take a few days. There is no way to know," he said. "Listen, before I leave with the group, I will help find you a place to stay tonight."

I looked around at the surrounding town. From what I could see, finding a decent place to stay was going to be a big problem. We finally found a roadside motel. The building was run-down. When I got to my room, the smell nearly knocked me over. Along the base of one wall, I saw cockroaches scurrying amongst rat feces. A single lightbulb hung down from a wire in the middle of the room. My attorney went to the room with me. "I think they will get this cleared up very quickly. You are no security risk. This is obviously a case of mistaken identity." He looked around the room and sighed. "Hang in there, buddy. It's just one night."

I smiled. "I've seen worse." After I got checked in, we found a small store where I purchased a toothbrush and toothpaste, along with a small bar of soap. I had $200 cash on me, along with a credit card. I did not have a cell phone with me. Back then, cell phones were not as prevalent as they are today. However, I had my attorney's number. I could call him with a phone card if I needed him.

My attorney and the rest of the group got in our van and went north to the border. I walked down the dusty main road to purchase a telephone calling card. Thankfully, every place in town accepted U.S. dollars as payment. I went to a local shop and bought some rice and beans and a bottle of Coke, along with a large container of bottled water.

Back in my room, I picked up the phone and called Prema. I told her everything that had happened. "Don't worry. Everything will be all right," I told her, even though I wondered if it would be. Then I called Father Carmen and told him what had happened. I asked him to pray and asked him to tell the reverend sisters at the convent to start praying as well. Finally I called my family in Nigeria. I had one request for them: pray! From across the globe, my prayer warriors went into battle, asking God to manifest Himself and make a way where there seemed to be no way. I knew our prayers would be heard: "For where two or three are gathered together in my name, there am I in the midst of them."[1] The people whom I asked to pray were all such holy people that I believed God was more likely to hear their prayers than mine, since I was such a miserable sinner.

After calling everyone I could, I tried to go to sleep. The pillows and bedsheets reeked. The awful smell kept me awake. Across the room, I could see the eyes of rats staring at me in the shadowy darkness. I turned the light back on. The rats scattered, as did the roaches. The night wore on. At about 10:00 p.m., the motel became noisy. I went out on the balcony of my second-floor room and looked down at the street below. A parade of men and women went in and out of the motel. As it turns out, the motel was full not only of rats and roaches but of prostitution as well. Part of the parade ended up in the rooms around me. The loud sound of people having sex echoed through my room. The stench of marijuana also hung in the air from the street below.

I felt trapped. I could not go out because the streets seemed like a dangerous place to go in the middle of the night in a country where I stood out. My fears rose up inside of me. With nowhere else to turn, I began to pray. I prayed every prayer I knew. After I went through all the prayers I had learned over the years, I started talking to God like one speaks to a dear, trusted friend. I poured out my heart and my tears to him. *O God Almighty, You have guided me from the shores of Nigeria to the mountains of America. You did not bring me into the middle of the sea to let me drown.* I prayed this over and over, weeping as I did. Finally the rooms around me grew quiet, as the sky outside began to brighten. Eventually, I nodded off to sleep, tired and overwhelmed.

At 9:00 a.m., I awoke with a start. I quickly brushed my teeth, washed my face, and ran off to the embassy in hopes of hearing some good news. When I walked into the embassy waiting area, the woman who had been so kind the day before motioned for me to come over to her window. "We have not heard back from the embassy in Nigeria," she said, "but I have talked to your attorney, and we sent a reminder to Nigeria. All we can do at this point is wait. I'm sorry."

I thanked her and left to go back to my hotel. Walking once again down the dusty streets of Nogales, I watched the hustle and bustle around me. Poverty surrounded me. The city lacked the basic infrastructure of even a small American town. Yet in the midst of the poverty, I noticed teenage boys and girls and young adults, all dressed like Americans. They wore the same brands and carried themselves with the same distinctive American swagger. The scene around me told me why the embassy had such a long line every day. People stood in line to get a day pass to go across the border to Nogales, Arizona, to go shopping. I wondered where they got the money to afford such expensive clothes and shoes.

On my way back to my motel room, I stopped at a store and bought more food and another calling card. *Surely tomorrow God will answer my prayer,* I thought. The one person I had not called the day before was my younger sister, Mie-Mie. She was an attorney who was working for Shell Petroleum in London at the time. She had just completed her PhD in energy law in Dundee, Scotland. When I heard her voice, I poured out everything that had happened.

"I know it looks dark, Bene, but be patient and do not panic. God will manifest Himself. You will see," she said.

"I hope you are right, but I don't know what I can do. There is no one I can call, no one I can contact. I feel trapped here," I said. I went on to explain how the problem was all the way back in Nigeria with the American Embassy there.

Mie-Mie had an idea. "Do you remember our friend Eddy? He is very well connected to the current Nigerian government. I will call him and see if there is anything he can do."

We talked a little longer. After I hung up, I went back out onto my balcony to watch the parade of people on the street below. However, on this my second night in Nogales, something was different. I noticed four men dressed in some type of security attire in front of the motel, as if they were standing guard. Right off, I could tell they were law enforcement officers, perhaps secret service. *Word must have gotten out that a possible Nigerian terrorist is in this motel*, I thought. One of the men turned and looked up at me. He stared at me until I became uncomfortable. I felt like they were there to keep an eye on me.

I moved back inside my room and decided to go to bed. First I washed my clothes in the sink. After two days, they were starting to smell. I also feared I would look even more suspicious if I appeared disheveled the next day. I lay down and tried to get to sleep. The light stayed on. I didn't dare turn it off because of the rats and roaches. The noises of the prostitutes and their customers echoed through the room once again, while the rats sat in their holes staring at me. My mind kept turning to the officers on the street below me. I wondered if they really were police officers. What if they were part of a drug cartel? At some point, I feared I could be killed in this motel and no one would ever know what had happened to me.

As my fears grew, I began to pray Scripture back to God.

"Even now I know that whatever you ask of God, God will give you," I prayed.[2]

"And whatever you ask in my name, I will do, so that the Father may be glorified in the Son. If you ask anything of me in my name, I will do it.[3]

"If you remain in me and my words remain in you, ask for whatever you want and it will be done for you.[4]

". . . so that whatever you ask the Father in my name he may give you.[5]

"Amen, amen, I say to you, whatever you ask the Father in my name he will give you."[6]

I prayed this all night. I prayed for my family and for Prema, because I knew they were in pain with worry over me. I prayed until I fell asleep in deep mental fatigue.

While I laid on the filthy bed in my rat- and roach-infested motel room, phone calls were being exchanged on the other side of the world. Mie-Mie called our family friend, Eddy. Eddy then called a close friend who was the secretary to the president of Nigeria, General Olusegun Obasanjo. When the secretary heard of my predicament, he placed a call from the office of the president of the Federal Republic of Nigeria to the United States Embassy and asked why an innocent Nigerian man's name had been placed on the security alert list.

This was not the first call to the embassy, but it was the first to which they paid attention. They had ignored the calls from the embassy worker in Nogales because I was a nobody to them. If they had not acted, I would have been deported from Mexico back to Nigeria. For those two extra days I was there, I was officially an illegal immigrant. But when the secretary to the president of Nigeria called the embassy, the staff sprang into action. Apparently, in the post 9/11 world, an embassy worker in Nigeria had gone over the names of those who had received temporary visas to the United States. Anyone he could not immediately trace, or anyone who had not checked back in with the embassy in Nigeria, was placed on the security alert list. I had checked in with an embassy every year when I went in to renew my visa. However, because I had not returned to Nigeria, an embassy worker in Lagos decided at whim that I was a security risk.

The president's secretary swept this misunderstanding aside and asked them to act swiftly to clear up my predicament. The embassy did. Again, I had no idea any of this was happening when I dressed in the morning and went back to the embassy in Nogales. The men outside the motel were gone when I walked out. The moment I walked into the embassy, I looked for the only woman I knew there. When I could not find her, I sat down on the bare floor because all the chairs in the waiting area were taken. The woman spotted me before I saw her. She came out into the lobby and motioned to me to come to her window. She smiled and asked, "How are you doing this morning?"

"Uh, so-so."

"I have good news that will brighten your day. Your name has been removed from the list. Here is your passport. The visa has already been stamped. You can go home now. Good luck."

If I could have, I would have reached through the bulletproof glass and hugged her. Instead I said thank you over and over. She was an angel to me, the only one in a very dark place. I then gathered all my papers and went out into the street. Before I could take another step, a wave of relief and joy swept over me. I sat down on the side of the road and wept. Passersby looked at me like I was a lunatic but I did not care. Once I gathered myself, I walked as quickly as I could to the border station. With every step I prayed, *Thank You, Jesus.* The border looked like the light of resurrection to me.

As soon as I stepped back into America, I found a pay phone and called my family in Nigeria. Through tears of joy, I said to them, "I am home now." Then I called Prema, and we cried together on the phone. I did the same with Father Carmen. He said to me, "Peace be with you, Bennet, and glory be to God. Come home." That's all I wanted to do as well. The cab ride from Nogales to Tucson and the flight back home to Pittsburgh cost me a small fortune, but I did not care. God had rescued me. I came away convinced that nothing is too difficult for Him. God will make a way where there seems to be no way. If you place your trust in Him, He will make the impossible possible. It was an invaluable lesson to learn in light of what I was about to face.

Chapter Fifteen

The NFL = Big Tobacco

My alarm went off at 3:00 a.m. the morning I set out to start writing my first Mike Webster paper, which was going to be the very first case study of Chronic Traumatic Encephalopathy in a football player reported in the medical literature. I took a quick shower to clear my head and sat down at my desktop computer. Then nothing happened. I stared at the screen, unable to force any words out. Once or twice, I managed to write a paragraph, but I immediately deleted it. None of the words I wrote sounded like what I wanted to say. It was very frustrating. Finally I gave up and went in to the office and lost myself in my work. I tried not to think about the paper.

The second morning, I woke up early, again, but just like the day before, I could not write anything worth keeping. The words I pecked out on the keyboard never formed a cohesive thought. This was very unusual for me. Mike Webster was not the first paper I had submitted for publication, nor would it be the last. In addition to writing academic papers, my job demanded that I write scholarly works on a regular basis for the courts or attorneys or Dr. Wecht. Never before had I struggled so much to put my thoughts into words.

When I had the same experience on the third day of writing, I knew this was more than a case of writer's block. Suddenly the cause dawned on me. My spirit whispered to me, *Bennet, give it a name.* I could not force words onto the page because I was trying to describe a condition and a disease that remained nameless. In a way, the lack of a name kept this disease detached and distant. It was like a stray animal that comes to the house. When the animal is just a cat or a dog, it annoys you and you try to get it to leave. The moment you give it a name, that animal becomes part of your family. The nameless condition I tried to describe was no different.

Okay, I need to give it a name, I thought to myself. *But what?* I spent the next two weeks contemplating that question. In my mind, the name had to meet four criteria. First, it had to be intellectually sophisticated. Second, it needed to have a good acronym, which would help it stick and make it more likely to permeate society. Third, the name also had to be generic enough to give me some wiggle room if my concepts were proven wrong and yet specific enough to actually describe the disease I had observed.

Finally, I recognized this was ultimately an occupational disease, and being an occupational disease, it was only a matter of time before it ended up in a court of law. As such, it had to fulfill what is known in the American legal system as the Daubert standard.[1] The Daubert standard states that for scientific evidence to be admissible in court, it must be a generally accepted principle and must have precedent. Therefore, I could not use any novel name I wanted, like dementia footballitica, because such a phrase had never been used in any medical literature.

My search for a name took me back to my original research. Going back to the time of Hippocrates, I identified thirty-seven descriptive terminologies that had been used to describe symptoms of permanent brain damage following blunt force head trauma. As I went through the list, two terminologies stood out above the others: Chronic Traumatic Encephalopathy and chronic traumatic brain injury. I quickly settled upon Chronic Traumatic Encephalopathy, or CTE. Chronic means "long term"; traumatic means "associated with trauma"; and encephalopathy means "a bad brain." In other words, the terminology referred to a bad brain associated with trauma over a long period of time. That was exactly what I had observed in Mike Webster. I now had my name.

I chose Chronic Traumatic Encephalopathy to fulfill the purposes I laid out for my criteria in finding a name. I believe my efforts were very successful. Fifteen years ago, no one had ever heard of CTE. Today, nearly everyone who watches or participates in football is very aware of it, even down to the little children in my son's kindergarten class. When I walk in the door of his classroom with him, the other students will ask me, "Are you the CTE doctor?" I believe that if I had used a totally novel name that had never been used in the medical literature, it would have made it easier for sports leagues to reject or deny CTE in the court of law based on the Daubert standard.

• • • •

Long before I sat down at my computer to write my paper describing CTE in Mike Webster's brain, a flood of research into the dangers of concussions and head injuries related to football was already in full swing. I thought I had discovered something new—and the brain disease I named CTE was, in fact, a new diagnosis. However, the fact that so-called *mild* traumatic brain injuries incurred in football and other contact sports can result in long-term, life-altering, and potentially life-ending problems was already well-known, at least to the National Football League.

Football has always been known to be a violent, dangerous game. Congress nearly banned it in the early twentieth century when a rash of players died on the field, many from head injuries. Back then, the game was even more savage than it is today. If not for President Teddy Roosevelt's intervention and his insistence that rules be changed to make the game safer, the sport might have ended in 1905. The changes that came as a result of Roosevelt's intervention made the game safer, but it did not make it safe. Many rule changes were made—changes such as eliminating mass formations during play, creating neutral zones between the offense and the defense, and increasing the yardage needed for a first down from five yards to ten yards. The number of player deaths and serious injuries dropped and the game lived on, but it never became safe.

Head injuries were a problem from the start. Back in the days before helmets, players ran the very real risk of suffering a fractured skull. The sport adopted leather helmets in response to this problem. It was rather interesting for me to learn that the first leather helmet to be worn in a football game was created by a shoemaker in 1893 for Cadet Joseph Reeves, who wore it in the Army-Navy football game. Cadet Reeves had been advised by a Navy doctor that he would be risking death or "instant insanity" if he took another kick to the head.[2] Obviously, a thin leather helmet offered very little real protection to the player, but it gave a sense of security that he had at least done something to protect himself.

Plastic helmets eventually replaced leather, and face masks were added in the 1950s to protect players' noses and jaws. Unfortunately, the helmet that was implemented to protect players quickly became a weapon. No longer in fear of breaking their heads open, players could hurl themselves at one another fearlessly. As players began to use their helmets as weapons, head injuries moved from the outside of the skull to the inside. Even today, even after rule changes designed to minimize concussions and head-to-head contact, you can hear the pop of helmets colliding with one another on every football play, as offensive and defensive players slam into each other at the line of scrimmage.

In the early, middle, and late twentieth century, many papers were published in the medical literature stating that football players at all levels suffered brain injuries while playing football, and sizable proportions of football players suffered persistent and prolonged symptoms, such as headaches, nausea, vomiting, impaired vision, changes in behavior, loss of memory, inability to concentrate on tasks, etc. Yet none of these papers made waves within the football community, including a position paper published in May 1957 by the American Academy of Pediatrics stating that any child who is twelve years of age or younger should not play high-impact, high-contact sports like football, wrestling, and boxing.[3] A 2011 paper by the American Academy of Pediatrics and the Canadian Paediatric Society reaffirmed this position.[4] Yet the game continued on as it had. Concussions and brain injuries continued to plague the game. We as a society chose to look the other way and keep silent in conformational cast of the mind and cognitive dissonance, because of our idolization of football. God remained number one; football became number two; and our children and their lives were relegated to number three. However, in the fullness of time, the light of the truth will shine upon us, in His time.

By 1994, the National Football League faced its most public brain and concussion crisis. Several of the league's biggest stars, including future Hall of Famers Steve Young and Troy Aikman, went down with concussions. Aikman's was so severe that he had no memory of the National Football Conference championship game in January 1994, the game that his team, the Dallas Cowboys, won to advance to their second straight Super Bowl. Merrill Hoge, a running back for the Chicago Bears, quit the game in the middle of the season after suffering his second major concussion in six weeks in October 1994. Many major news outlets, including the *New York Times*, ran front-page stories about football's concussion problem. *Sports Illustrated* ran a three-part series in its December 19, 1994, issue, which focused on head injuries in the NFL. Other media outlets spoke out about the dangers of football. Even Congress took notice and talked of investigating the sport.

In response to the crisis, the National Football League assembled a panel of doctors to study the problem of concussions and head injuries and to make recommendations on how to make players safer. The head of the committee, Dr. Elliot Pellman, was the New York Jets team doctor. He was also a rheumatologist, not a neurologist. Under Dr. Pellman's direction, the National Football League's Mild Traumatic Brain Injury (MTBI) Committee studied brain injuries for more than fifteen years and produced more than sixteen scientific papers, which were published from 2003 to 2009 in *Neurosurgery*—the official journal of the Congress of Neurological Surgeons and one of the most respected medical journals in the world. The first two papers actually received warm reviews. Both studied how concussions occurred and the kinds of hits that produced the most concussions among NFL players. However, neither looked at the long-term effects of concussions, nor did they explore any links to long-term brain damage.

The NFL's first two papers were initially submitted for publication on April 21, and June 10, 2003, and were published in October and December 2003, respectively. The third paper was actually submitted on the same day as the second, June 10, 2003, with the fourth paper submitted to the journal on November 11, 2003. This means that all the research for the first four papers was completed about the same time. The second two papers showed the NFL's concussion committee's true intention. Rather than focus on the possible delayed and persistent effects of brain injuries suffered while playing football, the NFL chose to collaborate with a sister multibillion-dollar industry, the helmet industry, to synthesize data, propose, position, and justify that helmets are the answer to brain injuries and concussions suffered while playing football. The propositional value would be to make us believe that helmets protect us and prevent head injuries in football. The game could then continue to thrive; more helmets would be sold; and the two industries would continue to make their billions in revenues and profits.

As expected, these NFL papers posited in no uncertain terms that concussions were extremely rare in the NFL. In their view, in the off chance that a concussion did occur, there was nothing to worry about, since it is the mildest form of traumatic brain injury. However, being the benevolent organization that they are, the NFL joined with helmet manufacturers to make the supposedly concussion-proof helmet. Of course, all of this is ridiculous. The actual scientific fact is that there is nothing mild about a concussion. The human brain suffers serious microscopic injuries from both concussive and subconcussive blows to the head. No helmet can prevent this damage, for no helmet can stop the brain from moving around and colliding with the inside of the skull at the moment of impact.

Yet, to the NFL, the so-called "concussion crisis" was not a crisis at all, for they were already at work to solve the problem. You need to remember that Mike Webster was never diagnosed with a concussion, at least not officially, and yet he suffered massive and permanent head trauma from both concussive and subconcussive hits. That is not the message the NFL wants us to hear. They want to make us believe that concussions are the problem. And if they can prove that concussions are mild and are extremely rare in football, then football must be safe. We can continue to watch and to play, and we will not have to worry about any long-term consequences. As we continue our love affair with the game, the money keeps on pouring in for the select few.

While the NFL's concussion committee worked to make it appear that football players are at no risk of long-term brain damage, they actually admitted in the fourth paper that subconcussive hits can and do cause long-term brain damage, at least for boxers. The committee wrote, "It is well accepted that chronic encephalopathy of boxers results from the accumulation of damage from multiple subconcussive blows to the head over a prolonged period of time, not the number of concussions sustained."[5]

They went on to say, "There was no evidence of chronic encephalopathy in this group of football players who had sustained a relatively small number of multiple concussions."[6] The authors did admit that some players demonstrated permanent postconcussion syndrome, but "they clearly did not have chronic encephalopathy such as that seen in boxers."[7]

In essence, what they were then saying was that repeated blows to the head in boxing caused brain damage, but repeated blows to the head in football did not. They made this claim even after players like Mike Webster were awarded disability payments by courts and the league's retirement board—after concluding that football caused their brain injuries. The NFL's official research team ignored this fact and instead concluded that football does not cause brain damage because the helmet provides enough protection to keep the brain unharmed.

As I always remind medical students and resident physicians when I teach them, medicine is not an absolute science like mathematics or physics. One plus one will always be an absolute outcome—two—but in medicine, it is not like that. Medical research can always attain a desired or expected outcome based on how you tweak your research parameters, what assumptions you make, what principles you apply, what methodologies you adopt, what cohort you study, and what error rates you apply. You may perform a research study and come up with one outcome; another person may perform exactly the same research, make subtle and barely noticeable changes in the scientific assumptions and principles, and come up with a completely different outcome. Medical research in the hands of a conniving mind is a very dangerous tool that can be misappropriated for all kinds of intents and purposes.

In their seventh paper, published in January 2005, the NFL put forth questionable data and concluded that when a professional football player suffers a concussion, which in their opinion is the mildest form of brain injury, the concussed player should be returned to play the same day he suffered his concussion. They further concluded that when a concussed football player is returned to play the same day or in the same game in which he suffered a concussion, his clinical outcomes *are better* and he has *less risk* of permanent brain damage than a player who is taken out of the game completely following a concussion! They claimed that these players do not show any increased risk of subsequently developing a prolonged postconcussion syndrome or any other type of brain injury, including a repeat concussion, second-impact syndrome, any bleeding inside the skull or brain, or brain edema.[8] To make matters worse, the research team recommended that the same standard should be applied to high school and college football players when they are known to suffer concussions. I am sickened to think of how many former players now suffer from irreparable brain damage because a team doctor followed this recommendation.

• • • •

One of the final research papers produced by the NFL's Mild Traumatic Brain Injury Committee reached the logical conclusion of the research their team carried out, beginning with its inception in 1994. The committee summarized its research with these words:

When the immunohistochemical results are extrapolated to professional football players, concussions result in no or minimal brain injury. Repeat impacts at higher velocity or with a heavier mass impactor cause extensive and distant diffuse axonal injury. Based on this model, the threshold for diffuse axonal injury is above even the most severe conditions for National Football League concussion.[9]

That is, the NFL concluded that concussions on the football field result in no or minimal brain injury. Even worse, their "research" determined that the forces generated in head-to-head collisions on the football field do not rise to a level capable of producing serious injuries. In other words, football is safe for the brain. There is no need to worry. Other papers in this series concluded that repeat concussions pose no risk of greater injury than a single concussion and that it is safe for a player who has been knocked out to return to play in the same game.

As of the time of this writing, these positions have changed in that players now must pass a rigid concussion protocol before they are allowed to return to play. However, as recently as March 2016, one of the most influential owners in the NFL, Jerry Jones, told the *Washington Post* that it is absurd to claim there is a link between football and permanent brain injury and the disease CTE. He said, "We don't have that knowledge and background and scientifically, so there's no way in the world to say you have a relationship relative to anything here. There's no research. There's no data."[10] Indianapolis Colts owner Jim Irsay equated the risks of long-term brain injury to taking an aspirin. In a March 27, 2016, interview he said, "I believe this: that the game has always been a risk, you know, and the way certain people are. Look at it. You take an aspirin, I take an aspirin, it might give you extreme side effects of illness and your body . . . may reject it, where I would be fine. So there is so much we don't know."[11]

All of this is completely and totally absurd. Any "research" that concludes concussions do not cause brain injuries flies in the face of two thousand years of accepted medical facts and common sense. The same is true of the National Football League's findings that players who have been knocked out can safely return to play in the same game without risk of further injury. Their research is very similar to studies produced by tobacco companies that claimed smoking is not harmful in any way. When you consider that the original head of the NFL's MTBI Committee was a rheumatologist, not a neurologist or neurosurgeon or neuropathologist, their conclusion makes a little more sense. I cannot even begin to describe how wrong both Jerry Jones' and Jim Irsay's statements are. To compare the risk of debilitating injuries like those suffered by Mike Webster—and many, many other players—to that of taking an aspirin is more than insulting to those whose lives have been permanently altered by the game. It is an outrage.

•　•　•　•

When I examined Mike Webster's brain in 2002 and 2003, I had no idea any of this so-called research was going on, for the papers had not yet been published. I did not know the National Football League was in the process of loudly proclaiming that the brains of its players were not at risk. "There is no danger here," they essentially said in response to the so-called concussion crisis. "There is nothing to see. Just move along." The NFL's response to concussion danger is very much like the cigarette industry's response to all the evidence of the dangers of smoking. Big Tobacco produced reams of "research" demonstrating how safe cigarettes are, even though knowledge of the dangers of smoking goes back to the days when tobacco was first discovered in the Americas. The 1999 Academy Award-nominated film *The Insider* chronicles the way in which the truth finally came out. In many ways it is quite similar to *Concussion*, although the message of *The Insider* is more easily accepted by the public.

The NFL had a more receptive audience to the research and message of denial. The millions of football fans in America—who each week engage in a form of conformational cast of the mind and of cognitive dissonance—find it easy to believe these super-sized men on the football field are indeed superhuman. These players overcome in weeks the kinds of injuries that would probably keep a normal person down for months or longer. As violent hits play out on the television screen, fans jump back and scream, "How can anyone get up from that?"—only to see players jump to their feet and run back into the huddle, ready for more. Even though fans' eyes told them no one could walk away from these "car wrecks" unscathed, conformational intelligence told them not to worry. The NFL's research told fans everywhere exactly what they wanted to hear: the game is safe and fun, and we can watch and enjoy without guilt. The players are fine. The games will go on. We should all sit back and enjoy.

Then I came along and found evidence of long-term, destructive trauma inside the brain of an NFL player. Why had no one ever found this damage before? There is only one reason: no one else had ever looked for it! No one wanted to know the truth! If they had, they would have discovered it years, perhaps decades, before I ever met Mike Webster.

Mike Webster was the first case, but as you will discover as you continue reading, he was not the last. Over the past decade and a half, more and more brains of football players have been studied, and CTE has been found to be widespread. And it is not only in the brains of football players, but in the brains of other athletes who play high-impact, high-contact sports like wrestling, ice hockey, boxing, mixed martial arts, and rugby. We do not yet know what percentage of people who play football and other high-impact, high-contact sports will develop CTE. I believe the percentage is very high. I firmly believe that O. J. Simpson has CTE, a topic I will return to later. Even though we cannot yet know exactly how many current or former players have CTE, since the disease can only be confirmed via autopsy, one thing is very clear: 100 percent of those who have ever played or ever will play football at any age are at risk of brain injury and permanent brain damage. One hundred percent. Not just professional football players, but anyone who plays football at any level. *All are at risk.*

This is why I am so adamant that children under the age of eighteen should not be allowed to play football or other high-impact, high-contact sports. Children should not play football, because the developing brain is especially susceptible to long-term damage from trauma. Studies have found the human brain does not fully develop until between the ages of eighteen and twenty-five. Why then would we expose the brains of our children to trauma?

We have laws against smoking until the age of eighteen or older. The legal drinking age is twenty-one. One could argue that smoking is actually safer for a child than football. I know that sounds outrageous, but hear me out. Smoking damages the lungs and leads to pulmonary and heart diseases, as well as greatly increasing the risk of cancer. Cigarettes shorten lives. Football-related brain disease, including CTE and PTE (Post-Traumatic Encephalopathy), takes away one's life even as the body goes on living, and it may eventually shorten one's life. I have met or heard from countless grieving mothers who have told me how their sons' behaviors drastically changed. These young men went from having energetic, intelligent, outgoing, vibrant personalities to being withdrawn and depressed. Men as young as the early twenties struggle to remember something as simple as where they live. They erupt in sudden outbursts of anger, becoming violent when they have never been violent before. To their family members, they look the same on the outside, but inside something has changed. The man they once knew is gone because his brain has been permanently altered.

The brain is where the mind resides, along with our intellect, our moods, and our emotions. Our brains define us as human beings. The core of our being rests in the 2.8 pound, semi-solid, Jell-O–like mass that rests in a liquid bath inside our skulls. When the mind goes, we cease to be. Shouldn't we then do everything we can to protect the most vulnerable among us—our children?

The most sinister aspect of CTE is the fact that the symptoms may not immediately manifest themselves. Damage done to the brain in the teen years may not reveal itself for years, perhaps a decade or more and even into one's forties. The damage shows up as memory loss; impulsiveness; diminished intellectual capacity; mood disorders, including depression and rampant fluctuations in mood; suicide attempts and actual suicides; changes in personality; increasing tendencies toward violence and criminal behavior; disinhibition; sexual improprieties and indiscretions; alcohol abuse; drug abuse; and exaggerated responses to life's daily stresses.

Every time I hear a news story of a former football player arrested for criminal behavior, especially domestic violence—and especially when this behavior comes suddenly, out of the blue—I suspect the cause can be traced back to head trauma suffered on a football field back in their days in Pop Warner football, high school football, and college football. Again, why would we expose our children to such risks?

. . . .

When I first started writing the Mike Webster paper, I knew this was where I would end up. I was beginning to realize how the NFL had tried to cover up this truth. By moving forward with the paper, I put myself on a collision course with the most powerful sports league in the world. They believed I would not survive. Over the course of the next few years, there were many times I thought they were right. If not for the grace of God and the strength given by the Holy Spirit, I would have given up the fight and my voice would have been silenced. Yet God sustained me. He gave me my resolve and my voice. God is the one who empowered me, because at its roots, CTE and sports-related brain trauma are spiritual issues. God loves His children and wants to protect us from harm. Shouldn't we do the same for our fellow human beings?

Chapter Sixteen

"In the Name of Christ, Stop!"

Early in the fifth century, an ascetic monk from the east felt compelled to travel to Rome, a city he had never visited before. He arrived to find huge crowds all moving in one direction. Since he did not know why the Spirit had led him to the city, he decided to follow the crowd. He quickly became caught up in the festive mood that permeated the crowds. His sense of expectation rose as the push of the crowds led him to the coliseum, where he sat down with the rest of the people and waited to see what might happen next. He did not have to wait long. Two gladiators came out into the arena and began fighting with swords and shields. Telemachus had never seen such a sight. Horrified by the sight, he stood on his seat and shouted, "In the name of Christ, stop!" No one paid any attention to him. The rest of the crowd cheered at the top of their lungs as the two gladiators began to draw blood from each other.

As the crowd cheered, Telemachus ran down from his seat and jumped into the arena. He went straight to the two gladiators, shouting, "In the name of Christ, stop!" The fighting men ignored him until he put himself between them. When the crowd saw him interfering with their entertainment, they began to boo and shout for him to get out of the way and let the show continue. Telemachus would not budge. "In the name of Christ, stop!" he shouted again. The crowd went from annoyed to enraged. A gladiator pushed Telemachus to the ground. As he lay in the dirt, the angry mob surged toward him. One man threw a stone at him, striking him in the chest. Another stone came flying in—and then another and another. He shielded himself with his arms, but the flurry of stones was too strong. Telemachus tried to get up from the ground but was knocked back down as a rock struck him in the head. A stream of blood spurted out. The blood only seemed to stir up the anger of the mob even more. "In the name of Christ, stop!" he said one last time. The stones continued to rain down, even after the small monk stopped moving. When it was clear he was dead, the anger of the crowd turned to revulsion over what they had done. Those who had cheered for blood felt very different when it covered their own hands. Saint Telemachus could not stop the gladiator combat show in the Roman Coliseum that day, but his death ultimately moved Emperor Honorius to ban the fights forever.[1]

I did not set out to be a modern-day Telemachus when I started writing my first CTE paper. I had not taken up the cause of telling the world, or at least America, the inherent dangers of football. At the time, the paper was nothing more than the final step to fulfill the promise I had made to Mike Webster, not a crusade.

This was not my first academic journal article. Around the time I started working on the CTE paper, another paper I had written came out in the *Brain Pathology* journal titled "Fatal Fulminant Pan-Meningo-Polioencephalitis Due to West Nile Virus."[2] The paper developed out of an autopsy I had performed on an eighty-seven-year-old gardener who died suddenly after three days of flu-like symptoms. As it turned out, his was one of the first reported cases of West Nile virus infection in a human being that originated in Pennsylvania. I was the lead author of a team of five. Four years later, I along with several others authored a second paper that studied six additional cases of West Nile virus.[3] Academic papers are an important part of the scientific process. As a physician, I have to self-finance and publish scientific papers, if and when I can, to do my own little part to advance medicine and improve our lives. I also authored four papers that explored a possible link between bariatric surgery and suicide. Writing the two West Nile virus papers did not mean I had taken up the study of the disease as a life's cause, any more than exploring the link between bariatric surgery and suicide meant I hoped to become the expert in that field. The CTE paper was more of the same.

As I wrote in the last chapter, the hardest part of writing the paper was getting started. Until I came up with a name, words refused to come. Once I settled on CTE, the words seemed to fly out. I completed the first draft of the paper in a little over a month. While I made multiple revisions based on editorial input from my coauthors and the editors at the journal that published it, the bulk of the paper is the same as that original draft. I truly believe my writing was guided by God Himself. Right around the time the movie *Concussion* was released, I went back and reread the CTE paper for the first time since its publication. To be honest, I nearly fell over when I read it. *This came out of me?* I thought in amazement. *This paper is too good to have been written by me!* I was floored by its audacious scientific originality, creativity, and innovation.

The Bennet Omalu of today could not write such a beautiful piece. At that time, I was still filled with youthful idealism and hope. When I wrote that paper, I believed it would truly make a difference, that it would spark a genuine dialogue within the football community that would result in a game that protects its players. I boldly spoke my mind and made the type of strong assertions Dr. Wecht had taught me to make whenever I spoke as an expert in a court case. My boldness was based on truth. I had no reason to be anything but forthright. I did not take a side in the paper. Truth does not have a side. Truth is truth. It is up to us to conform to truth; truth does not conform to us.

The paper focused on one case—that of Mike Webster. My co-authors and I included photos of the slides of his brain that showed the tau proteins. While the paper focused on Mike, I included information I discovered regarding the frequency of concussions in football and other contact sports. The paper acknowledged the research that had been done up to that point while calling for further study of the long-term, chronic symptoms of brain injury in retired players. I wrapped up the paper with this conclusion:

This case study by itself cannot confirm a causal link between professional football and CTE. However, it indicates the need for comprehensive cognitive and autopsy-based research on long-term postneurotraumatic sequelae of professional American football. Empirical, cognitive, and postmortem data on CTE are currently unavailable in the population cohort of professional NFL players. Our report therefore constitutes a forensic epidemiological sentinel case that draws attention to a possibly more prevalent yet unrecognized disease because of the rarity of CNS-targeted autopsies in the cohort of retired NFL players.[4]

In laymen's terms, the above says that Mike Webster is probably not an isolated case, that many more former football players probably suffer from CTE. However, because there had not yet been a concerted effort to look for the presence of CTE in the brains of former football players, we have no way to know how widespread this disease might be. I assumed many of those connected with football would be anxious to know more, since I also assumed they surely had the players' best interests at heart. Yes, I was young and very naive.

After completing the first draft, I set the paper aside for a short time and then went back and made revisions. I sent copies to Drs. DeKosky and Hamilton, along with Dr. Wecht. I also sent a copy to Ryan Minster and Ilyas Kamboh, both of whom were in the Department of Human Genetics at the University of Pittsburgh. These men were my coauthors on the paper. Each of them suggested changes. Some I accepted, while some I did not. I sent the final draft back to them all. We went back and forth until we had a manuscript we were all proud of.

Now the question was where to submit the finished paper for publication. I believed there was only one logical choice: *Neurosurgery*, the same publication in which the NFL concussion committee presented its research. The journal's editor at the time, Michael Apuzzo, was a professor of neurosurgery at the University of Southern California. Under his direction, the journal had added a sports section that featured articles on sports and the brain. Since *Neurosurgery* had already published NFL papers focusing on football and concussions, it seemed the logical place to submit my paper.

I printed out several copies of my paper and mailed them to Dr. Apuzzo in August 2004. The journal required several copies, since every submitted paper goes through a process of peer review. Typically, the paper goes to two reviewers. If they agree a paper is publishable and meets the ethical and generally accepted medical standards, the paper is published. If the two disagree with one another, a third reviewer is brought in to break the tie. Many times the reviewers will make recommendations for revisions or clarifications, which the author must make. All of this is done under the supervision of the journal and section editors. The whole process is a rigorous intellectual back-and-forth that can take months to complete. In the end, however, it should make the paper even stronger.

From what I observed in the review process, I believe my paper went through many reviewers—possibly up to eighteen—not two or three. Why so many? I do not know. All of them sent comments to me. While many were positive and asked legitimate scientific questions that I needed to clarify, others had a decidedly negative tone. Many of them did not want to see my paper published, but the reasons they gave were not scientifically valid. Some of the negative comments questioned my credentials. They insinuated that I was a no-name and a quack. *Who is Omalu?* they essentially asked, *and why should we take seriously the research conducted by nothing more than a government employee doing autopsies in Pittsburgh?*

The attitude expressed by these reviewers speaks to one of the fallacies of accepted scientific research. Today, the scientific community yields to established, experienced professors in university settings to guide research, review research papers, and determine whose research is funded. The result is a complete lack of innovative approaches to old problems. Instead, we are stuck with conformational intelligence, where the same approach is used over and over. We need a new model of funding research that targets young researchers with out-of-the-box, nonconformational thinking hypotheses and concepts that may not belong or want to be within the four walls of a university, especially in this era of emerging virtual research. If I had done my research in a university setting, I believe I would have been told to stop.

Looking back, I wonder if my story might have a different ending if I had approached a different journal with my CTE paper. I did not know it at the time, but it seemed that *Neurosurgery* was becoming the official voice of the NFL regarding brain injuries. One of the first NFL's MTBI papers published in *Neurosurgery* was accompanied by a guest editorial by the then NFL commissioner Paul Tagliabue. Tagliabue is a lawyer who was paid millions of dollars each year by the NFL owners to maximize profits for the league. Michael Apuzzo also penned an editorial announcing the NFL's series of papers. In it, he compared professional football to the Roman gladiator contests, with all of their splendor and pageantry. Apuzzo had a front-row seat to that pageantry, since he had worked as a consultant to the New York Giants and was with them when they played in the 2001 Super Bowl against the Baltimore Ravens.

The seemingly endless process of back-and-forth with the many reviewers left me very frustrated. I suspected that none to several of those reviewing my paper were trauma neuropathologists. Many of their comments made it clear they may not have been adequately educated on the pathology of neurotrauma. The process of answering their questions and objections took three to four times the amount of time it took to write the paper itself. My responses were more than five times the length of the paper. Yet no matter how much I wrote, more questions came.

My patience began to wear thin. Gradually, without my knowing it, a simmering anger arose within me. I could not believe this was happening in America. In all fairness, some of the reviewers were good to me and commended me for my work. A minority remained vehement that the paper should never be published and that Omalu should not be trusted because his assertions are dangerous.

However, to the credit of Dr. Apuzzo, *Neurosurgery* ultimately decided to publish my paper. They included some of the comments from reviewers, but most of those included were positive. One in particular stood out. Dr. Donald Marion, a neurosurgeon from Boston, gave some very constructive comments. Given what happened next, he was an angel from God to me, encouraging me when I could have easily drowned in a sea of doubt.

Finally, I received a copy of the volume 57, number 1, July 2005, issue of *Neurosurgery*. I opened to page 128 and just stared at the article. I did not reread it. I had read it enough times during the editorial process. Instead my thoughts turned to Mike Webster and his family. *You've been vindicated, Mike*, I thought. *After reading this, people will know you did not want the life into which you descended. Football did that to you. I hope this gives you rest.*

And then I closed the journal and set it on a shelf. I never could have imagined that this was going to be deemed one of the most influential case reports in sports medicine. When I closed the cover of *Neurosurgery*, I did not imagine that paper would come to define so much of my life and my life's work. In my mind, it was very much like the other papers I wrote both before and after Mike. I had discovered something in the brain of Mike Webster and now I had reported it. That afternoon I went back to work and completed another autopsy then filed my reports on it, just as I did every day. The Mike Webster paper was just another day at the office, not a life-defining moment.

Then the NFL stepped in.

One morning several weeks after the publication of "Chronic Traumatic Encephalopathy in a National Football League Player," my phone rang. Dr. Wecht's secretary was on the phone. She only called when there was a problem or when Dr. Wecht needed me. As expected, she said, "Cyril needs to reach you. May he call you at this number?" she asked.

"Of course," I said.

A few minutes later, the phone rang again. "Bennet," Dr. Wecht said in an anxious tone of voice. He was usually very loquacious, but not this morning. "I just got off the phone with an editor from *Neurosurgery*."

"Is everything alright?" I asked.

"No. The NFL sent them a letter demanding that your paper be retracted. They want you to say you made the whole thing up."

I sat there stunned for a moment. "What did the editor say to them?" I asked.

"Dr. Apuzzo has set up a review committee to address their concerns and determine if it should be retracted."

I wondered if this had been the original plan all along—if they had only agreed to publish my paper to embarrass me. Now it made sense. By holding me up to professional ridicule, they would send a message to other doctors across the world that you don't mess with the National Football League. If my paper was retracted and all my science debunked, then my career was as good as done. No one would ever touch me or the question of CTE ever again. Panic started to set in—panic and anger. But then I remembered the words of Saint Paul:

> We know that all things work for good for those who love God, who are called according to his purpose . . . If God is for us, who can be against us? . . . What will separate us from the love of Christ? Will anguish, or distress, or persecution, or famine, or nakedness, or peril, or the sword? . . . No, in all these things we conquer overwhelmingly through him who loved us. For I am convinced that neither death, nor life, nor angels, nor principalities, nor present things, nor future things, nor powers, nor height, nor depth, nor any other creature will be able to separate us from the love of God in Christ Jesus our Lord.[5]

Once I calmed down, I realized I had the least to lose from this battle. My coauthors were far more established than me. I was only three months out of my training as a neuropathologist when I conducted the Mike Webster autopsy. I was a neophyte. But Drs. Wecht, DeKosky, Hamilton, and Kamboh had their names and reputations on the line. I wondered if they regretted becoming associated with this no-name Nigerian doctor.

"So what should we do, Cyril?" I asked.

Dr. Wecht laughed. "Don't worry about these idiots," he said. He actually used a much more colorful term, which is Dr. Wecht for you. "Don't let them intimidate you or silence you. Dr. Marion is going to call you later. Listen to him, and do whatever he asks you to do."

"I will," I said. I hung up the phone and whispered to myself, *What have I done?* Tears rolled down my face. I knew I had done nothing wrong against anyone. Everything I had done that led up to this moment, from ordering the fixing of Mike Webster's brain to the extensive study of the slides of his brain to all of my research into brain disease and ultimately in publishing this paper—all of it was driven by my desire to have justice for Mike and restore his humanity. And now I was under attack. My career and the careers of those who had stood with me were all at stake. I knew what I had to do. I had to stand firm on the truth. Truth will not be moved or intimidated by those who seek to silence it.

I had never set out to become a modern-day Telemachus. My goal was never to be the voice of an outsider who points out what no one else was able to see because their eyes were clouded by conformational intelligence. If the NFL had simply ignored my first paper, I may never have become the one running out into the football arena and crying out, "In the name of Christ, stop!" But once they demanded a retraction, that was exactly who I became. I had no choice. I had to be the voice for those who could no longer speak for themselves. And the next voice that needed to be heard came to me very quickly.

Chapter Seventeen

The Baton Is Passed

Terry Long joined the Pittsburgh Steelers in 1984 when he was drafted in the fourth round out of East Carolina University. In Pittsburgh, players are not just drafted by the team; most are adopted by the city, at least while they are with the team. Terry played for the Steelers for eight seasons. By his second season, he was the starting right guard, where he lined up right next to Mike Webster. The two played together through the 1988 season. Mike finished out his career in Kansas City, where he played two seasons. Terry remained in Pittsburgh, a fixture on the offensive line until injuries finally ended his career after the 1991 season. When his playing career came to a close, he stayed in Pittsburgh. It had become home.

On June 7, 2005, several weeks before my paper appeared in *Neurosurgery*, Terry Long was found unresponsive in his home. Apparently, he drank a large amount of antifreeze and took his own life. He was forty-five. I was not on duty when his body came to the coroner's office. Dr. Abdulrezak Shakir conducted the autopsy. When he removed Terry's brain from the skull, he did not see any abnormalities. He did not cut the brain; rather, he paused. "I wonder if Bennet will want to examine this?" he asked the others in the room. The consensus was to fix the brain and save it for me. When I came into work the next Monday, I walked into the autopsy room, and everyone yelled, "Dr. Omalu, we have another brain for you—another NFL player!"

That is how I met Terry Long.

After the brain became fixed in formalin, I took possession of it and examined it by myself at the medical examiner's office. I took slices from different regions of his brain and packaged them so that slides could be made from them. After my Mike Webster experience, I knew exactly what to look for across his brain. Unlike with Mike, I did not wait weeks and months before examining the slides for evidence of CTE. Between the time of Terry's death and the preparation of the slides, I received the letter from the NFL demanding that I retract my first paper. When Terry's brain cells showed the signature CTE patterns of tau proteins and other changes, I knew that not only was I not going to retract my first paper; I was looking through the microscope at my second.

Before I started the paper on Terry Long, which I titled "Chronic Traumatic Encephalopathy in a National Football League Player: Part II," I had to respond to the NFL's criticism of the first paper. And the criticism had been harsh.

Dr. Donald Marion was the one who called and explained the situation to me. In that phone call, he spoke in a calm but affirmative way as he explained the implications of what was going on. "The NFL's concussion committee has demanded a retraction," he said, "and the editorial board is going to consider their arguments to see if they are valid." My heart sank a little. "However," he continued, "I don't think every doctor who disagrees with a paper should request that it be retracted. That's not good science. Periodicals like ours provide a platform for debate. Both sides may present their data, and ultimately the truth will prevail. We put your paper through a rigorous peer review process, and we felt the scientific basis of the paper was sound. That's why we published it."

"So what do I do now?" I asked.

"I will fax the NFL's letter to you. You'll have two weeks to respond. Then we go from there."

"Thank you," I said, more than a little relieved.

"Do you have any questions?" Dr. Marion asked.

"No, sir, I don't," I said.

"Good. Now listen, Bennet, I don't want you to get down or feel rushed. All I'm asking is that you understand the seriousness of the situation and respond accordingly. Focus on the science. Don't attack on a personal level. Review your data, and let it speak."

When I sat down to write my response, that was what I tried to do. However, as hard as I tried, my emotions came through. I could not help myself. The letter demanding my retraction came from Drs. Pellman, Casson, and Viano, all members of the NFL's Mild Traumatic Brain Injury Committee. While Dr. Casson is a neurologist, Dr. Pellman is a rheumatologist, and Dr. Viano is a biomechanical engineer who did crash-test studies with dummies for General Motors. None were neuropathologists, and yet they found fault with my neuropathological work. The bulk of their reasoning came down to this: I claimed Mike Webster's problems came as a result of head trauma he suffered from playing in the NFL for seventeen years. However, they said I failed to show a medical history of trauma. In my paper, I wrote that Mike Webster had no known history of brain trauma outside of professional football. In their counterargument, they responded, "In fact, there was no known history of brain trauma *inside* professional football either."[1]

When I read that line, I nearly fell out of my chair. I asked myself, *Have they ever even* watched *football?* Former Pittsburgh Steelers Craig Wolfley, who was a left guard next to Mike Webster while Terry Long was at right guard, described playing in the NFL to the *Pittsburgh Post-Gazette*. "'I used to laugh when people would ask what's Sunday like,' he said. 'I would say, well, you get about six inches from a brick wall and you ram your head into it about 75 to 100 times. Ha, ha, ha. Well, it's not so funny years later when you realize it's consistent trauma.'"[2]

What was obvious to the players on the field was apparently not obvious to these leading researchers of the great and mighty National Football League. Dr. Pellman worked on the sidelines in NFL games. How could he have missed the violent collisions taking place in every play? *How is this happening in America?* I wondered.

Prior to focusing on Mike's history of brain trauma, Drs. Pellman,

Casson, and Viano argued that the accepted form of traumatic enceph-alopathy is that found in boxers—dementia pugilistica or punch-drunk syndrome. Because Mike Webster did not demonstrate the same symp-toms, he obviously did not have dementia pugilistica and therefore did not have CTE. Yet that was exactly the point I had made. Of course Mike Webster did not have dementia pugilistica, simply because he was not a boxer, and his brain did not show the changes we would expect to see in a brain with dementia pugilistica. The patterns of tau proteins, amyloid proteins, and other changes spread across Mike's brain were consistent with a new condition—CTE—and also consistent with the pattern of impacts a football lineman encounters throughout the course of an ordinary game and a career. I wondered if these men had even read my paper, since they built one of their primary arguments on a point on which we both agreed.

After reading the letter, I became so upset that I had to sit down and calm myself. Once my heart rate was back to normal, I wrote out my response. Although I tried to keep emotions out of it, that proved impossible. Thankfully, my coauthors edited out much of the emotion-alism. We came away with a reasoned response that Dr. Marion found sufficient. The response letter had some humor in it. In a way, I prodded my critics and suggested they were idiots, but I didn't come out and say it in those terms. I basically said these guys cannot be serious. If you read the letter, you will understand what I am talking about.[3]

In the end, Dr. Marion rejected the NFL's call for a retraction. In fact, he also penned a response to the NFL's letter, which appeared in the May 2006 issue of *Neurosurgery*, alongside the NFL's letter and my group's response. I am very thankful for his thoughtful response to the critics of my paper. Just as he urged me to do, Dr. Marion focused on the science. He upheld my methods, but he did more than that. In his final paragraph, Dr. Marion chided the tone of the Pellman group's letter. Dr. Marion wrote, "As members of the Mild Traumatic Brain Injury Committee of the NFL, and clinician-scientists that are clearly devoted to the inves-tigation of sports-related concussion, Drs. Casson, Pellman, and Viano should welcome the contribution from Omalu et al. and consider the findings of that report highly relevant to their own research, rather than recommending retraction of the article."[4] I felt both validated and free to investigate fully the new case before me—that of Terry Long.

• • • • •

In life, Mike Webster and Terry Long had been teammates. Mike was the established veteran when the Steelers drafted Terry. When Mike left as a free agent and signed with the Kansas City Chiefs for his final two seasons, his mantle passed to Terry. In death, they worked together once again. Terry took up the baton from Mike in the relay race for the truth. Just as I felt Mike's spirit urging me on, I felt the same from Terry.

With Mike, I went public with my findings in the *Neurosurgery* paper. After I told Dr. Wecht that I had confirmed Terry had CTE, the second definite case, he decided to go public right away. Dr. Wecht held a news conference in which he told reporters that Terry Long had the same brain disease as Mike Webster, and that disease caused him to kill himself. News outlets all across America ran variations of the headline that appeared in the *Pittsburgh Post-Gazette*: "Wecht: Long Died from Brain Injury: Had Head Trauma from NFL Days."[5] More than a decade later, a headline like this has unfortunately become all too common, as CTE is found in the autopsies of former players ranging from Hall of Fame legends like Frank Gifford to those who had barely gotten started in the league, like former New York Giants safety Tyler Sash, who died at the age of twenty-five. However, in 2005, this was huge news that shook the football world, especially in the Midtown Manhattan headquarters of the National Football League.

The counterattack began the day after Dr. Wecht's claims went public. Longtime Pittsburgh Steelers neurosurgeon Dr. Joseph Maroon called Dr. Wecht's claims about Terry Long "preposterous and a misinterpretation of facts" and "fallacious reasoning."[6] Dr. Maroon had been with the Steelers since 1981. He was there when both Mike Webster and Terry Long played. Other NFL doctors chimed in. Some suggested that what I was doing was not science—or at least it was questionable science. They dismissed me as a dangerous human being who should not be trusted. Reading between the lines, I saw an insinuation that I was a foreigner who was attacking an American way of life. I started receiving phone calls, many of them filled with threats, either blatant or implied. More than once, I noticed cars following me as I drove. They did not try to hide the fact that they were tailing me.

The office where I worked had also been rocked by unexpected news. An investigation by the FBI led to a grand jury indictment of Dr. Wecht on eighty-four counts that all came down to alleging he used the county's government resources to benefit his private consulting company.[7] Dr. Wecht was forced to resign, although he had done nothing wrong. I was called as a witness against him. It was like testifying against my own father—that is how close I felt to Dr. Wecht. The case dragged on for three years before finally coming to trial in 2008. In my testimony, I tried my very best to say good things about Dr. Wecht, like a son would say of his beloved father, to let the jury know that in front of them sat a very good man who had been very good to me and made me who I am. All the charges against Dr. Wecht were later dismissed by the court, but by then, the damage was done.[8] Neither of us remained in the medical examiner's office by the time he was cleared. I had moved on to California—but I'm getting ahead of myself.

The storm of criticism leveled at me after we announced that Terry Long had CTE stirred up a fire of anger inside me. The NFL's researchers had criticized my first paper for not including enough of Mike Webster's medical history. I decided to apply my role as a forensic pathologist to CTE. When crimes are committed, I do more than examine the body; I go out and conduct postmortem interviews with family members and social contacts. I decided to do the same with my CTE cases.

Even though I had finished my work with regard to Mike Webster, I began with his family and friends. His son, Garrett, told me about both the good times and the bad with his father. He helped me understand the frustration the family felt in their inability to help Mike. I also spoke with his ex-wife, Pam. She said something I was hearing over and over again from the families of other players: "Bennet, if you had only come sooner before Mike died. I did not know how sick Mike was. If I had known, maybe I could have helped him more."

One interview not only helped me understand Mike; the man I interviewed became a lifeline for me. Bob Fitzsimmons had been Mike Webster's attorney for several years. As I spoke with Bob, I quickly realized this was a man I could trust. We developed a friendship. Bob became my attorney, adviser, mentor, and friend. He is one of the angels God placed in my life to help me survive the storm that my discovery of CTE unleashed. Bob had already fought the NFL on behalf of Mike, suing the league for disability payments for the head trauma Mike suffered while playing. More than three years before Mike Webster died, Bob had already started the campaign to prove that football had permanently altered Mike's brain. In the process, Bob became one of the few people in the world Mike completely trusted in the last few years of his life. I soon learned why. I feel the same way.

Because of his own battle with the NFL, Bob was very sympathetic to my struggles. He also offered me hope, because he had gone up against the NFL's toughest lawyers and won. On October 28, 1999, the NFL's disability board admitted that football had damaged Mike's brain. However, even then, the board refused to grant the full amount that Bob was seeking for Mike. That prompted Bob to file another suit, all of which was a precursor to the class action suit brought against the NFL by more than five thousand former players.[9] Bob was not intimidated by the NFL, and he saw it for what it was. In his own fight for justice for Mike Webster, he had gone up against many of the same people who were now criticizing me, including Dr. Maroon, the Steelers team neurosurgeon. Dr. Maroon said that making the claim that football had damaged Mike's brain was highly questionable.[10] Incidentally, Dr. Maroon was one of the doctors who devised imPACT (Immediate Post-Concussion Assessment and Cognitive Testing), the most widely used neuropsychological exam, which they assert helps determine when a player can return to play after a concussion. The test is used even though the FDA has stated that imPACT cannot be used for the diagnosis of a concussion or to determine appropriate treatments for a concussion.[11] Every sports league on every level—from youth leagues to the professionals—uses imPACT. However, I am very doubtful of a test that supposedly protects the brains of players when it could not protect the brains of the players on the team where the test was first developed. To put it simply, imPACT does not play any role in preventing or improving brain damage after an athlete has suffered a concussion!

Through all of this, Bob Fitzsimmons and I bonded. We are still close friends to this day.

After interviewing Mike's friends and family, I went to see Terry Long's family. Family members told me how Terry changed toward the end of his playing career. He had become depressed and attempted suicide for the first time in 1991, at the beginning of his last season with the Steelers. After his playing career ended, he jumped into one risky business venture after another, taking huge risks that invariably failed. He increasingly became a very scared and paranoid man. His wife, Lynne, told me he had huge mood swings. He jumped from being kind and gentle to being hostile in a matter of moments. In time, he became more and more withdrawn, locking himself in his house for days to avoid all outside contact. Lynne said the same thing Pam Webster told me: "Why didn't you come sooner? I didn't know he was sick. Maybe I could have helped him." Her words broke my heart.

I included the details of Terry's life in the second paper. My reasons were twofold. First, I wanted to disarm the critics of the first paper who said I did not include enough of Mike Webster's medical history. Second, I wanted to show the kind of man Terry Long was. While the paper was titled "Chronic Traumatic Encephalopathy in a National Football League Player: Part II," this NFL player was more than a statistic; he was a man.[12] Including details of his life was my way of affirming his humanity as a child of God. This was not just a football player whose life had been cut short by brain trauma suffered while playing football; this was a son and a husband, a kindhearted man who funded a scholarship at his alma mater.

I submitted the paper to *Neurosurgery* in January 2006. The same team came alongside me as coauthors. Dr. Abdulrezak Shakir, the pathologist who conducted Terry Long's autopsy, also contributed to the paper. Surprisingly, in June of that year, *Neurosurgery* agreed to publish after the usual back-and-forth with reviewers. The paper appeared in the November 2006 issue. Two months earlier, the NFL had published Part 13 of their research into concussions. Their paper declared that new football helmets with thicker, more energy-absorbing padding were the answer to the concussion problem.[13] They weren't. This was yet another systemic and systematic ploy of the NFL to misappropriate medical science, either by fault or default, and thus mislead the public.

One month after the second paper was published, my home phone rang. Prema answered. Another former NFL player had died. The caller, Chris Nowinski, asked if I could help get consent from the family to have the brain examined for CTE. I did not know Chris well at that time, but I agreed to help him. The player, Andre Waters, had died in Tampa, Florida.

This was not the first time Chris had called my house. Over the previous few months, he had called multiple times and left messages about a book he was writing. I did not know who he was, so I was not interested in his book. Sometimes in our lives, our spirits guide us to do or not to do something for reasons we do not really know or understand. I think the Spirit was guiding me away from Chris. But after many calls and messages, Prema, who did not want to hear any more of his messages, firmly asked me to receive his call and speak to him. I did. Given the way things played out with Chris, I should not have, but that's another story.

A few weeks later, I was on a plane to Florida. Tests revealed that Andre Waters did indeed have CTE.

At this time, I had taken possession of the residual, formalin-fixed brains of Mike Webster and Terry Long. An attempt was made by some detractors to destroy the brains. The technician who was asked to secretly destroy them called me and advised me to obtain written consents from the families. She did not think such valuable brain specimens should be destroyed. This technician proved to be another angel in my life.

I was now examining these brains on my balcony in my condo. Prema secretly took pictures of me examining these brains, for she wondered what a weird man she had married, a man who examined human brains at home. But I had to do what I had to do, since no institution or university in the United States of America offered me any platform to continue my work.

Andre Waters became the third confirmed case of CTE, and in the world of medical science, three cases are not a coincidence. It is a precedent and a trend. I immediately planned on writing a third paper. This time, I believed that those who had dismissed my research would have to take notice. Mike Webster and Terry Long were not outliers. I believed we had just touched the tip of the iceberg.

Unfortunately, word got out about Andre in a way over which I had no control. The news that Andre Waters had CTE did not break on the pages of *Neurosurgery*. Nor did it become public through the Allegheny County medical examiner's office to the *Pittsburgh Post-Gazette*. Instead, the story broke on the front page of the *New York Times*. On the morning of January 18, 2007, the newspaper ran this headline: "Expert Ties Ex-Player's Suicide to Brain Damage."[14] Chris Nowinski gave the story to his close friend—freelance reporter Alan Schwarz. As soon as the *Times* ran that front-page story, football-related brain trauma and CTE went from a debate held on the pages of a medical journal to a national topic of conversation everywhere, from the halls of Congress to the family dinner table.

At the time, I thought this would be a good thing. I believed the debate would result in more research into brain trauma and contact sports and change the way in which football and other games are played. In my naiveté, I still thought this news would be welcomed by football and, even more, by America.

I was wrong.

The Baton Is Passed

The *New York Times* story unleashed a storm of attacks unlike anything I had ever experienced before. I had awakened an angry sleeping giant and the object of his wrath was me, Omalu—the little man from a faraway land who dared threaten the giant's greatest love. I found myself pulled into a fight I could not win. I only hoped I could survive it.

Chapter Eighteen

Marginalized, Minimalized, Ostracized

O nce the Andre Waters case went public, I realized I had no other choice but to go deeper in my research of CTE. Up to this point, I had worked on purely a case-by-case basis. I'd found the disease in the brains of three former NFL players, but I knew they would not be the last. The disease needed to be studied with the goal of finding a cure.

Before I discovered football through Mike Webster in a city whose life and dynamic revolve around its professional football team, I never could have imagined that the idea of preventing a disease like CTE by avoiding contact sports could in any way be considered controversial. For me, it seems like common sense. If you do not want brain trauma, avoid head trauma. What could be simpler? However, common sense is not common in the face of conformational intelligence. When I say, "Avoid sports and activities that involve repeated blows to the head," people hear me say, "Football is bad, and football is evil." That is why I knew I needed to go deeper in my research of CTE.

My mind was filled with questions about this disease. I wanted to study retired players, especially the living members of the football Hall of Fame, to find out how many of them displayed symptoms associated with brain trauma. Since head trauma is not limited to football players, or even to athletes, I wanted to expand the study group to include those who played other contact sports, as well as members of the military. While CTE can be presumptively diagnosed in the living based on a constellation of symptoms and signs, CTE can only, like Alzheimer's disease, be definitively diagnosed through an autopsy after death—at least at the time of this writing. Therefore, I wanted to try to develop a test that can definitively diagnose the disease in the living. Once we can identify and quantify CTE in the living, the next step is to develop a cure.

The size and scope of the research I wanted to undertake went well beyond what any one individual could achieve in a lifetime. Therefore, I began reaching out to others to be partners in research. I began with the place I knew best—the University of Pittsburgh Medical School and School of Public Health. I failed to mention earlier that I earned a master's degree in public health, with a focus on epidemiology, at the university, in addition to my fellowships in forensic pathology and neuropathology. The university and I knew each other well. Some of the leading neurological researchers in the country were on the faculty. I was a part of the two schools as adjunct faculty as well. It only seemed natural to reach out to key department chairs and directors of research programs with the goal of establishing a program at the university to research CTE. I assumed the university would embrace me as one of their own and provide seed money for research, as well as laboratory space and personnel.

I identified four key men to approach with my idea. I met with each individually and explained what I wanted to do. The meetings could not have gone worse. One man never even made eye contact with me. Within five minutes, I was heading out the door. Two of the others looked me in the eye and made it clear they had absolutely no interest in what I proposed. The fourth, a neurosurgeon, was the nicest to me. He listened thoughtfully. At the end, he told me two things. First, he advised me to avoid the press. Then he told me he would get back in touch with me. He never did.

By this point, Dr. Wecht had left the Allegheny County medical examiner's office. He resigned in January 2006. His replacement was, unfortunately, very familiar to me. He had been the county forensic pathologist in the Thomas Kimbell case. The fact that my testimony had called his work into question in that case did not exactly endear me to my new boss. The first three months my new boss was on the job, he barely acknowledged my presence in the office. Even worse, he took a stance on my work with CTE that was opposite Cyril's. One day I went looking in the office for the files connected to the cases of CTE. The files and slides were missing. I asked around the office, but no one knew what had happened to them. Finally I learned that my new boss questioned my conclusions, so he sent them to other doctors across the country to review my work. While peer reviews are a good thing in medicine, this was not a normal peer review. One of my former neuropathology professors alerted me that my boss had come to him looking for faults in my work. My new boss had already made up his mind that I was not to be trusted as a doctor and a scientist. I could see the writing on the wall. It certainly looked like he was trying to find a way to get rid of me. Between work and the university, I felt like a persona non grata—a nonentity, a person of no consequence. As I read my Bible, I came across a story about persons with leprosy who were ostracized by everyone.[1] I knew how they felt.

Never one to take a hint, I kept moving forward in my search to further research into CTE. Dr. DeKosky agreed to write a letter to the National Football League and to the NFL Players Association (NFLPA), proposing a joint research project. We included the players' union because it should be most interested in protecting the health and well-being of its members. Dr. DeKosky proposed a longitudinal study whereby we would follow, monitor, and study four hundred NFL Hall of Famers, the cream of the crop. In addition to looking for and monitoring any symptoms they might have while living, their brains would be examined for evidence of CTE after their deaths. I asked Dr. DeKosky to write the letter, because he is a well-known and respected neurologist and one of the leading Alzheimer's disease researchers in the country. The NFL had already closed their book on me, but they should have been open to this proposal from Dr. DeKosky. After several months went by without a response, we sent a follow-up letter. We're still waiting for a response to this day.

• • • •

Even without any partners stepping forward to join me in my research, I continued my own efforts to learn as much about the disease as I could. To be honest, simply identifying the disease as a result of an autopsy left me sad, frustrated, and angry. The next phase of my research took me out of the lab and more deeply into the lives of the players who had suffered with the disease. My old depression returned, because the stories I heard broke my heart. My faith in America began to be shaken.

Andre Waters' story especially touched me. His mother—a single mom with eleven children—told me the story of her son. Life was hard for the family when Andre was a boy. He used to go with her and work in the cornfields to help put food on the table. Football gave him the hope of a better life. A star high school football player, he received a scholarship to a small college in Philadelphia. He signed with the Philadelphia Eagles as an undrafted free agent and went on to play twelve years in the NFL. His all-out style of play earned him the nickname Dirty Waters because he hit so hard. For his mother, Andre's making it to the NFL was an answer to prayer. A descendant of slaves, the entire family saw Andre's achievement as an opportunity to rewrite their family's history and grab hold of the American Dream. Andre bought his mother a new house and car and asked her to quit working. She didn't.

Andre's mother never knew the toll the game was taking on her son. After his fifteenth concussion, he stopped counting. His playing career ended in 1995. That was about the time family members noticed that Andre was becoming forgetful. At first they thought he was just absent-minded. Eventually, he had to call family members and ask for directions when he became lost on familiar roads on his way home. His personality also changed. Andre became very isolated, some days never even getting out of bed. Mood swings and exaggerated responses to minor events left people around him feeling like they were walking on eggshells. He went downhill from there until he took his own life.

When I returned home from meeting with Andre's mother, I sat down and cried uncontrollably. The pain was too much to bear. Andre and his family saw his NFL career as a way out of the abject poverty they had known in the past. It seemed their family history had been transformed from its roots in slavery to laying hold of the American Dream. This is one of the greatest fallacies of professional football. Fans believe the players all become fabulously wealthy and leave the game set for life. In truth, the median NFL player's salary is less than one million dollars a year.[2] While that seems like a lot, keep in mind that out of their salary, they must pay their agents a percentage, while their union fees take another cut. Then they have to pay taxes. After deducting all the taxes and fees, the player is left with something closer to $300,000. The average NFL career is 3.5 years, and most players are out of the game by their thirtieth birthday. That means the average player earns about $1 million in take-home pay over his career in the NFL.

And what did they have to give up for that payday? Emerging studies are suggesting that more than 90 percent of the brains of football players show CTE changes when they die. In one such study of thirty-five professional football players, only one—a twenty-six-year-old man—did not show any CTE change.[3]

Personally, I have yet to examine a brain of a professional football player who did not have CTE. The only negative case I have found was that of a twenty-four-year-old football player, whose partial brain was sent to me in small sections. However, I believe if I had examined his whole brain, it would have been positive for CTE. The fact is, if you play football at every level, especially beginning as a child, you have a 100 percent exposure risk to permanent brain damage. I do not believe CTE will affect every football player or players of other high-impact, high-contact sports to the same degree. But the absence of incapacitating symptoms does not mean there is no CTE pathology or other evidence of brain damage, at least on the cellular level. Sometimes the degree of observable pathology in the brain does not correlate with the degree of symptoms one may suffer. We observe the same phenomenon in other types of dementias.

NFL players put themselves at risk, even though they are among the lowest-paid professional athletes in comparison to the other major sports. The average Major League Baseball salary is $4 million. The average National Basketball Association salary is just under $6 million. Even the average salary in the National Hockey League, the least popular of the four major American sports, tops the National Football League average.[4] Of those four, only football and hockey are high-impact, high-contact sports with a high risk of brain trauma. Some will still argue that even though NFL players earn less than athletes in other major sports, they still make a lot more money than the average fan does. That is true, but that argument also overlooks what takes place after football. A 2009 *Sports Illustrated* study found that nearly 80 percent of NFL players were either bankrupt or under financial stress because of joblessness or divorce within two years of leaving the sport.[5] If only their minds could heal as quickly as the money disappears.

• • • •

Andre Waters' mother's stories made me want to know more about him. I took time off from my job and took a red-eye flight to a Southern state to meet his niece, with whom he lived the last few years of his life. I rented a car at the airport and took off driving toward the town where she lived. In those days, I never thought anything about driving anywhere late at night. I often took late flights so I could leave after my workday was done. However, I had never driven in the South before.

It was well past midnight when I pulled into a rural gas station. When I walked in, the black man behind the counter gave me a look that made me want to laugh. In a deep Southern accent, he said to me, "Boy, where are you off to at this time of night? You gotta be outta your mind to be driving this late."

"Why?" I asked.

When he heard my accent, he did a double take. "Where you from?" he asked.

"Pittsburgh," I said.

"No, where you from? That ain't no Pittsburgh Yankee accent."

"Nigeria," I said.

"Well, son," he said, adding extra syllables to each word, "you may not understand what I'm fixing to tell you, but it is dangerous to be driving around these parts at this time of night all by yourself as a black man. Now you may not get what I'm saying, but you don't need to be taking no unnecessary risks."

"I'll stay safe," I said. I wasn't making an empty statement. I felt safe because I felt the presence of the Spirit of Almighty God with me. Not only that, but I felt the spirits of Mike Webster, Terry Long, and Andre Waters riding along with me. This was their fight. They were going to protect me.

I made it to my meeting with Andre's niece. Her stories also shook me and left me grieving over what the game of football took from him. When I left the next day for the long drive back to the airport, her stories kept running through my mind. At one point, I had to pull over because my tears were clouding my vision. The thought of Andre Waters—and who knows how many other players suffering in obscurity and in total silence—broke my heart. When they played and gave everything they had on the field, crowds cheered, and people treated them like royalty. Fans in the stands wore jerseys with the players' names scrawled across the back. But once they were too broken-down to play, they were dropped like sacrificial lambs. The fans moved on to the latest set of players. When stories like Andre Waters' suicide made the news, the fans stopped for a moment and uttered things like, "what a waste!" and "he had so much going for him"—and they went right back to cheering for their team, oblivious to what their favorite sport had done to their heroes. That's what made me so angry and upset. Once the great heroes could no longer perform, they were forgotten.

Meanwhile, the NFL doctors began referring to me with all sorts of adjectives across all media. They made it sound like I was a dangerous human being who could not be trusted, an outsider, a foreigner who was attacking the American way of life. Then phone calls started coming to the house—threatening calls. I did my best to ignore them, but I could see the toll they were taking on Prema. This wasn't the life she anticipated when she married me. We had started work on our dream house in a beautiful neighborhood in suburban Pittsburgh, a project Prema and I began before the storm over CTE came. Before we decided to build, we tried to buy a home in an exclusive neighborhood. The deal fell through, mysteriously. We later learned we would have been the first black family in the neighborhood. The realtor implied that it was the reason the seller had changed their minds about us.

The phone calls grew more threatening. People told me to go back to the jungle where I had come from. They threatened me and my family. I then started noticing cars following me. And I wasn't just being paranoid.

The worst came one morning when I had to drive up to Buffalo to the Canadian consular office for a Canadian visa interview so I could go to the U.S. Embassy in Canada to renew my U.S. visa. I got into my car at 3:00 a.m. As I put on my seat belt, I noticed a brown Crown Victoria sedan parked across the street. When I started my car, the lights of the Crown Vic came on. We were living in a condo. As I pulled out of the condo parking lot, the car pulled right behind me. It stayed behind me as I drove down toward the freeway, and then it followed me onto the freeway ramp. I exited from one freeway to another. The brown car matched me turn for turn. I felt like this was a movie, and I was on the wrong side of a car chase.

A half hour went by. The brown Crown Victoria sedan stayed right behind me. It had dropped back a little to appear less conspicuous, but at this early hour, hardly any cars were on the road. The longer the car stayed behind me, the more scared I became. I didn't dare pull over out of fear that they might walk up to me and shoot me. My ears became tuned to any strange sounds from my car. For all I knew, they might have done something to it to cause me to crash. I kept my speed slow, around 50 miles an hour, for fear that they might try to ram me and make me crash. Honestly, I had no idea who these people were and why they were behind me, which made my mind jump to every possible bad conclusion. After receiving so many threatening phone calls, I think anyone would have done the same.

The car stayed behind me. *Well, if this is it, this is it*, I thought. *Jesus, I love You. All I have is Thine. Yours I am, and Yours I want to be. Do with me what Thou wilt.* Over and over, I repeated this prayer. Finally, after about thirty minutes, the car exited off of the freeway. I took a deep breath and started singing a Nigerian spiritual song as loudly as I could. "We are saying thank You, Jesus, thank You, my Lord. We are saying thank You, Jesus, thank You, my Lord." I kept singing until I exited.

My father called me a few days after this incident. "Bene, I have heard about what you are doing, but I want you to recognize that these are men and women who are invested in the affairs of this world, who are less likely to be afraid of God. Their God is the money they make, so you need to be careful. These are people who may not hesitate to harm anyone who threatens their revenue stream, and you should just be careful and trust God. Surrender all to Him, for He has led you thus far, and He will lead you on." My father was not asking me to stop doing what I was doing. But he did remind me that the strongest man is not the one who throws the first punch. It is often the man who chooses to walk away. I thanked my father for his advice, but I knew I was not going to walk away from my brothers who were suffering in silence and obscurity.

I did, however, decide to do something just in case something happened to me. I packaged all of my research and wrote a book, which I self-published, titled *Play Hard, Die Young: Football Dementia, Depression, and Death.* The book included profiles of Mike Webster, Terry Long, and Andre Waters. Before the book went to press, I hired a professional editor to clean up the prose and a publicity expert to promote it. We approached publishers as well, but they all turned me down. One publisher actually called me and told me he liked my book. But he said he didn't think any publisher would touch it because of an unspoken fear of the NFL. It reminds me of one of my favorite lines from the movie *Concussion*, when Cyril Wecht warns me against going up against a corporation that owns a day of the week. Eventually, I went ahead with self-publishing, a venture that cost me more than $50,000.

• • • •

While all of this was going on, another tragedy occurred. World Wrestling Entertainment professional wrestler Chris Benoit killed his wife and son in his suburban Atlanta home and then killed himself. Some had called Chris the greatest professional wrestler of all time. This tragedy shocked everyone who knew him and his family. The act seemed so out of character. No one saw it coming. Autopsies were conducted on the three bodies. The pathologist examined Chris's brain and then placed it back in the truncal cavity of the body. Sometime later, Chris Nowinski contacted the family, who granted consent to examine Chris's brain for evidence of CTE. I flew down to Atlanta to retrieve the brain and bring it back to Pittsburgh for examination. Because Chris had been dead for several days and his brain was mildly decomposed, I did not want to ship it via FedEx or UPS and risk causing further damage. Chris Nowinski met me in Atlanta. We picked up the brain, rented a car, and drove 700 miles back to Pittsburgh with the brain in a bucket of formalin in the back of the car.

When I got back home, I placed the bucket and the brain in a closet to allow it to fix thoroughly. The onslaught in the press against me intensified. To be honest, I began to wish I had never met Mike Webster. Lying awake at night, I wondered why I had ever ventured into this battle. I wanted to walk away. I wanted to go back to doing my job as a forensic pathologist and neuropathologist and get back to living my life. Outside of this mess, I had a wonderful life. Prema and I were building our dream home. We had a baby on the way. Life could not be better in every way except one. And that one was getting worse every day.

Several weeks later, I placed the brain of Chris Benoit into the back-seat of my Mercedes and drove to Morgantown, West Virginia, where my friend Dr. Julian Bailes invited me to use the autopsy room in his hospital to examine the brain. My heart wasn't in this examination like it had been in the previous three. But since Julian was nice enough to join me in this effort, I had to go through with it. The two of us got to know each other in the middle of the string of bad press and threatening phone calls. He called my office one morning and said something very few people had said: "Bennet, I believe you." For a neurosurgeon and former team doctor for the Steelers to say this meant a lot to me. I am deeply grateful to Julian, for at this time in my life, he was yet another angel of God who gave me a voice when I had no voice.

That is why, even though all of these events were starting to take their toll on me, I followed through with bringing Chris Benoit's brain to Julian. Together, we examined the brain, snapping pictures and taking samples. We finished around 6:30 in the evening. I carried the brain and the sections we had taken for histological analysis and staining back to my car. When I walked up to it, the left back tire was flat. I called the Mercedes Benz emergency road service. Forty minutes later, the technician arrived to assist me. "Hmmm, that's weird," he said.

"What?" I asked.

"The puncture is in an odd place. It's on the side. I don't see many punctures there," he said.

I didn't think much of it. He put the donut spare on, and I drove back to Pittsburgh. The hour-and-a-half trip took me more than two hours because I had to drive much slower with the small spare. By the time I got home a little after 10:00 p.m., I was frustrated and annoyed and just in a bad sort of mind. Prema was already in bed. She went to bed early most nights because she was pregnant. As soon as I got home, I went straight to bed myself. It had been a long day. I was ready for it to end.

The next thing I heard was my wife yelling at me to come to the kitchen. Startled, I had no idea what day or time it was. I stumbled out of bed and went to the kitchen. The clock on the microwave read 3:18. "Why did you start the dishwasher?" Prema asked.

"What?" Her question didn't make any sense to me.

"The dishwasher is running. It woke me up. When I opened it, I found it was completely empty. Why did you turn on an empty dishwasher?"

"Uh, I didn't," I replied. I reached over and switched the dishwasher off. Then I stood there for a moment, thinking. First I'd had the weird flat tire. Now I had this weird appliance episode. I spoke out loud, but not to Prema. "Look, Chris, I get it. I get it. I will not quit. I will do the best I can to help, but you folks have to help me and guide me. I promise I will do the best I can, but we have to work together as a team and fight this battle together, okay?"

Prema and I went back to sleep. We did not experience any other strange occurrences. Even so, a few weeks later, I moved Chris Benoit's brain—along with the remains of Mike Webster's brain, Terry Long's brain, Andre Waters' brain, and Justin Strzelczyk's brain—from my coat closet to Dr. Bailes' laboratory at the West Virginia University Hospital.

Chapter Nineteen

I Wish I'd Never Met
Mike Webster

My phone rang one evening. I recognized the number as an attorney friend of mine—an assistant district attorney. We didn't have any cases on which we were working together at the time, so I wondered why he might be calling. When I answered, he was quite upset with me. "Bennet, I thought you told me you discovered CTE. How could you lie to me?"

"What are you talking about?" I asked. "How did I lie?"

"I'm watching television right now, and there is a woman from Boston University on the screen who says she discovered CTE. Why would you tell me you discovered it if she did?"

I was so shocked that I could hardly speak. "Who is she?" I asked. My friend told me her name. I had never heard of her. Then he told me the names of a couple of other people in the same news report. I recognized their names as people who had at one time partnered with me, Bob Fitzsimmons, and Julian Bailes to do research on the extent of CTE. Bob, Julian, and I had later parted ways with them. "They're lying," I told my friend. I briefly explained who these people were and how the break with them had come about.

After hearing my story, my friend became even angrier, but not at me. He seethed. "Oh my God, Bennet, you know what they are doing, don't you?" he said.

"Taking credit for my discovery," I said.

"There's far more to it than that. You may not have grown up in this country, but there is a historical precedent to what they are trying to do to you. They want to replace your black face with that of a blonde-headed white woman with whom they are more comfortable," he said.

"How can this happen in America?" I asked.

"I don't know," my friend said, "but it does. Things like this happen all the time. If there is money to be made—either through a product or through gaining research grants and then marketing the results—there's a risk of this sort of theft of intellectual property."

As sad and dark as my attorney friend's assertions may seem, his assertions were confirmed several years later by the book and PBS documentary *League of Denial*. According to the book and documentary, the blonde white woman who claimed she discovered CTE was actually handpicked by Chris Nowinski and a man named Robert Stern from Boston University to examine the brains of football players after the Chris Benoit case and before the Tom McHale case. After my diagnosis of CTE in Tom McHale, a request was made by a family member for me to share the samples of the brain tissues with researchers at Boston University, and as a true scientist, I did so. But this group at Boston University went public with the results without giving me any recognition or acknowledgment whatsoever. To them I did not exist. Tom McHale was the first case of CTE in a football player announced by this group at Boston University.

When I hung up the phone, I muttered words I had begun saying a lot: "I wish I had never met Mike Webster. I wish someone else had been on duty the day he came into the autopsy room. I wish I had never fixed his brain and never had slides made and never looked at those slides under a microscope. I wish I had never started down this path that now consumes my life. I wish I had never met Mike Webster."

But then I remembered that Mike Webster probably wishes he had never met me. I'm sure he wishes he had picked a different occupation, one in which he did not receive blows to the head over and over again, blows that robbed him and his family of himself. And I am sure Terry Long wishes he had never met me. I am sure he wishes he could reverse time and choose basketball or baseball or building houses or anything other than football as a career. The same is true of Andre Waters, Justin Strzelczyk, Chris Benoit, Tom McHale, and every person on the growing list of those I had tested who died from causes related to CTE. Not one of them wanted to die young. Not one of them wanted their brains to betray them and turn them into a person they did not recognize. I wish I had never met Mike Webster, and the feelings were surely mutual.

But God had brought us together. Just as Mike had suffered, now I had to go through a different type of suffering—one of humiliation and the loss of everything I had spent a lifetime building. Within six years of meeting Mike, I had lost my job, my dream house, and nearly my place in this country. My friendship with the man who was a second father to me, Cyril Wecht, was severely strained—I feared beyond repair.

There were days I told myself that if I had not found CTE in the brain of a former NFL player, sooner or later someone else would have. I tried to convince myself that if I had walked away from Mike, someone else would have taken up this cause and incurred the wrath of the NFL, its researchers, and the list of organizations and agencies in whom the NFL had its hooks through the funding of research. This other unknown researcher could have gone through the professional suicide I had to endure, not me. *Why did it have to be me?*

But then I remembered the promise I had made to Mike. And I also reminded myself that the reason no one else had discovered CTE is no one else looked for it, in spite of the large number of former players struggling with brain trauma–related symptoms. That's why God chose me as a servant, as an outsider who did not think like everyone about football and those who play it. God brought me and Mike Webster together. I could not deny this truth, even as I wished He had chosen someone else.

• • • •

The woman on television taking credit for discovering CTE was just the latest in a string of humiliations that have continued to this day. They began with the NFL concussion committee's researchers demanding I retract my first paper. I should have expected their response. The powers that be reacted in the same way to the earliest studies that exposed the truth about dementia pugilistica in boxers, back when boxing sat atop the American sports scene. Doctors employed by the boxing industry systemically and systematically denied that boxing caused brain damage. I read one paper where a doctor with ties to the boxing industry claimed that boxing was no more dangerous than cycling or baseball.

While such a claim is obviously ridiculous today, people back then took it seriously. They did so because of the conformational intelligence of that day. Millions of boxing fans called it the "sweet science," which overlooked its brutality. At the time, it was one of America's favorite sports. When you are member of a group, the group influences your mentality, your presuppositions, and therefore your way of thinking and processing information, without you even being aware of it. You reach the same conclusion as the rest of the group, even when that conclusion is not supported by science. This occurs over and over with physicians connected to the sports industry. They become so intoxicated by the status, fame, and exclusivity of their connection to their sport that they become zombies without even realizing it. As someone who stepped in and observed this from the outside, I have thought this to be an interesting phenomenon.

The NFL medical researchers who attacked my research had the same conformational intelligence distort their perspectives. I do not know how else to explain how a member of the original NFL Mild Traumatic Brain Injury Committee, a neurologist with impeccable credentials, could go on national television and repeatedly insist that football causes no long-term risk of brain trauma. They denied my research, and even when they found they could deny it no longer, they denied me and my role in it. In the first conference the NFL convened to explore the long-term risks of brain trauma to players and the risks of CTE, they invited everyone to come and speak except me, even though I discovered the disease. They did not want to do anything to lend any legitimacy to me. To them, I am still today a nonperson they wish would just go away.

Yes, I expected the NFL to continue their efforts to humiliate me. I did not expect the same treatment from my colleagues who had no ties to the NFL. Before my first paper on CTE appeared in *Neurosurgery*, I presented it at an international meeting of the American Association of Neuropathologists (AANP). Even before presenting my paper, my experience with the AANP had been less than welcoming. I am not accusing the AANP of anything; I am simply stating my experiences and my perceptions from those experiences. When I went to an AANP meeting as a young neuropathologist, no one even extended the courtesy of talking to me, even when I initiated the conversation by saying hello. At one meeting I was standing by myself waiting for a conference to begin. One of my colleagues walked up to me and said, "Somebody spilled water on the floor over there. We need to get it cleaned up before someone slips and falls."

I looked at her with a very confused look. After several moments of awkward silence, I said to her, "I am a doctor here for the same meeting as you."

"I'm sorry," she said. "I thought you were part of the housekeeping staff." I've always wondered if this woman would have made the same assumption if I were white.

When I presented the Mike Webster paper, the AANP's reception was cold. I stood in the display hall next to the scientific poster of Mike, but no one asked me a question or commented on my research. Other doctors around me spoke of me in the third person as they stood right next to me as if I were not even there. Most of those who came by did not say anything with their mouths, but their body language spoke volumes. I felt very alone and very unwelcome, like an alien in an association of which I was a member. Not surprisingly, like an alien, I looked very different from everyone else in this meeting.

That was my last time to attend an AANP meeting. Nearly a decade and a half has passed since I discovered CTE, a subject that has advanced neuroscience and has brought the work of neuropathologists into the international limelight. It should not surprise you to learn that the AANP has never invited me to give a talk about CTE to share my experiences and perspectives. That is not to say they have not had meetings to discuss CTE. They have had many. Yet they have never once asked the neuropathologist who discovered the disease to speak. Even after the release of the movie *Concussion*, they have continued down this path. They regularly issue press releases promoting other members of the association as the leading authorities on CTE, but they rarely mention me by name.

I've received the same treatment from the National Institutes of Health (NIH), a federal agency set up by the government of the United States of America. This is the agency the nation trusts to lead the way in biomedical and health-related research. Even though the NIH has been very involved in brain trauma and CTE research the past several years, they have never reached out to me or even acknowledged my existence. Over the years, I have applied to them and other affiliated organizations for grants for my research, but I have always been turned down. Why? I do not know. Apparently my reputation at the NIH is not good. A close friend of mine, a fellow African, called me one day very distraught after attending a meeting with an NIH executive. My friend told me that the executive said she did not trust "that African doctor"—that is, me. She did not know me. She had never worked with me. She had never even talked to me, and yet she had already made a decision about my competence. My friend urged me to go public with the story, but instead I entrusted this battle to God. He knows the truth, and His truth will prevail.

Not surprisingly, it has been revealed that part of the NIH's funding for CTE research comes from the National Football League. In my opinion, I do not believe officials of the NIH or the Food and Drug Administration (FDA) should serve in any capacity on committees of organizations and corporations like the NFL and pharmaceutical companies. And when they leave the NIH or FDA, they should not be allowed to serve on such committees or work in such corporations until after five years.

The humiliation from the NIH was not just in the distant past. In 2015, I received a call from a very good friend of mine—a well-established and successful attorney. He said, "Bennet, have you seen the news today?" I said no. He told me the NIH put together a panel of neuropathologists from across the country to identify the neuropathological criteria for the diagnosis of CTE. He said he expected to see my name on the top of the list, but he scanned the list and did not see it. He asked if I had not been invited to the panel. I said no, that I was not even aware that the NIH was putting together a CTE panel. He was very upset and said that we could not stand by and continue to let this happen in the United States, that this was a very big slight to me. He wanted to do something. Again, I remembered that God fights my battles for me. I told him not to worry about it—that I have seen worse, and it did not bother me. Besides, I did not want to be part of a conformational group of neuropathologists. Where were they when I was discovering CTE? Many, if not all, of the members of that panel were the same members of the AANP who had excluded me. Some of them were the ones who continue to deny that I discovered CTE. I consoled my friend, and he calmed down before we hung up. I teased him, talked about other injustices in America, and hung up on a lighter note.

After I hung up, I had the same thought I have had so many times about not meeting Mike Webster. I would have been left alone. I could have just led my quiet life of faith and enjoyed the simple things of life. But God had other plans.

In spite of the treatment I have received from the AANP and the NIH, others have embraced me. Along those lines, I must give great credit to the College of American Pathologists, the American Association of Physician Leadership, and the American Medical Association, all organizations of which I am also a member. They have embraced me and my work, in spite of what others have said about me. I respect them very much, for they have treated me with dignity and respect—dignity given not because I am black or white or green, but because of the science behind my research and the impact of my research. That is the way it should be.

The NIH was not the only government entity that acted as though I had nothing to do with the discovery of CTE. Around the time the NFL held the conference to which they did not invite me, the Congressional Judiciary Committee held a public hearing to look into CTE, which was organized by Michigan congressman John Conyers. This hearing was the first of its kind. The commissioner of the NFL was called to speak, as were some doctors from Boston University. One of Congressman Conyers' assistants contacted me to formally invite me to the hearing. However, two days before the very highly publicized meeting, the same assistant called to tell me my invitation had been rescinded. He had no explanation when I asked why.

After I hung up the phone, I sat down and wept. *Even the United States Congress is ostracizing me*, I thought. *Why? What have I done?* It seemed like, since I was not yet an American citizen, I had nothing to contribute. This just struck me as contradictory to everything I ever believed about America. We are a nation of immigrants. Everyone came from somewhere else. I was not yet officially a citizen, but I was on the pathway to citizenship. I loved America, and yet this made me feel very much like the feelings were not mutual. Let me be clear: I do not think this was purely an anti-immigrant stance. Instead, I believe that in the hearts of those who made the decisions about the congressional hearing, my presence would have made everyone very uncomfortable, because I had essentially forced this situation on Congress. Bennet Omalu, a newly arrived American, had called into question the most American of sports—the sport that is intertwined into the culture, society, and identity of America. As Alec Baldwin (playing Julian Bailes) said to Will Smith (playing me) in the movie *Concussion*, in America "God is number one," which he said while holding up two fingers, and "football is number two," holding up one finger.

I also believe a large measure of my being shunned came because I had embarrassed those who should have discovered CTE long before I ever conducted Mike Webster's autopsy. The leading neurological and neuropathological researchers in the best academic and research centers in the country did not discover something that should have been very obvious for at least as long as football players wore plastic helmets and turned what should have been a piece of protection into a weapon. When I discovered the tangles of tau proteins in Mike Webster's brain, I was just three months out from completing my fellowship in neuropathology. No one with so little experience should have made such an important discovery. Discoveries like this should be made in the finest research hospitals and universities by middle-aged men with decades of experience. It seemed that the discovery by someone like me embarrassed them, and if I were to be invited to come to their hearings and meetings, my very presence might have reminded them of how they were failing the players they proclaimed to love and admire. No one wants to feel that level of discomfort. It was easier for all involved to pretend I did not exist, to render me a nonentity.

• • • •

The problems with the AANP and Congress and the NIH and all the rest were just beginning in 2007, which proved to be a very, very difficult year. Dr. Cyril Wecht had been indicted the year before and had subsequently resigned from the Allegheny County medical examiner's office. In the last chapter, I wrote about the difficulties I had with his replacement. As time went on, the tension in the office grew more pronounced. Finally I knew I had no choice but to resign my position. This decision placed me in a difficult spot. I had long since started the process of working toward becoming a United States citizen. That had been my goal from the time I arrived in Seattle. I fell in love with America from the start, especially after I moved to New York and experienced the wonderful diversity that makes America what it is. In spite of our flaws, this is still the place where people are the most free to pursue God's perfection within them and to become whatever we want to become. Where else but in America could my story be told, along with the stories of scores of others who have experienced the American Dream here?

However, I still had many years left before I met the residency requirements that would allow me to become a citizen. For me to maintain my visa, I had to have a job. When I quit the medical examiner's office in Pittsburgh, the clock started ticking. If I did not find a job in six months, I would be deported with no hope of returning. Up to this point, I not only had continued to work; I had also continued to pursue every educational opportunity I could reach for. My father had preached to me the power of education, and I took his words to heart. While in Pittsburgh, I completed two fellowships, earned a master's degree in public health, and another master's degree in business administration from one of the top business schools in the world—Tepper School of Business at Carnegie Mellon University. I eventually earned five board certifications in five subspecialties of medicine. I was busy.

However, all my work would be for naught if I did not find a new job. Resigning from the medical examiner's office was one of the hardest decisions of my life. Prema and I were building a nice life here. Work on our "million-dollar dream home" was nearly complete. We were expecting our first child. Prema had finished her education and had opportunities to work if she wanted. Life had come together for us in Pittsburgh. We were living the American Dream. But now everything was in doubt.

And then one of the worst moments of my life happened. I was at church on a Saturday morning getting the sound system ready for a funeral service. The matriarch of a prominent African-American family in Pittsburgh had passed away, and her funeral Mass was at St. Benedict the Moor. The church was going to be full, and many important persons would be attending the Mass. Father Carmen counted on me to take care of so many things. My phone rang, and it was Prema. She sounded distraught on the phone. "What's wrong?" I asked.

"I'm bleeding," she said.

I dropped everything and rushed home. I picked her up and took her to the closest hospital's emergency room. In a short time, our worst fears were confirmed: She had a miscarriage. I was devastated, not just because we lost the baby, but by Prema's pain. I did not want to see her suffer. She is such a lovely, reserved, down-to-earth person—simply an angel. To see her sobbing broke my heart. I wept too. Prema did not deserve this. I held her and promised her that it would be okay. God will bless us with another child very soon.

After a couple of hours, the hospital released us, and we went home. I called a close friend to come and assist us since we had no family in Pittsburgh. It was just Prema and me. I sped back to church to make it on time for the funeral Mass. We could not let Father Carmen and the mourning family down. We had to be there for them. During the Mass, I prayed that the Holy Spirit would descend upon Prema and grant her peace in this time of trial. She was too good a person to suffer this pain. God answered our prayers sooner than we expected. To Him be all praise.

Chapter Twenty

Finding Life
in the Wilderness

On August 17, 2007, Prema and I said good-bye to the city we had grown to love and good-bye to the dream home in which we would never live, and we moved as far away as we could from everything connected to football and the NFL. I had accepted the position to become the new chief medical examiner of San Joaquin County, California. I almost missed out on the opportunity. Several unsolicited calls came to me in Pittsburgh from a Captain somebody from a funny-sounding place in California. Since I did not recognize the name or the number, I ignored the call. So many angry phone calls came to our home that I had grown weary of even picking up the receiver. That might have been the end of it if a friend and colleague, a man who served as a resident under me while I was a fellow in neuropathology at the University of Pittsburgh Medical Center, had not called. "Bennet, a guy from California is trying to reach you. He says he has called you many times, but you do not return his calls."

I immediately became defensive. "Oh, do you know this guy?"

"Yes, Bennet. I'm the one who gave him your number. He wants to hire you," my friend said.

"Hire me? For what?" This shows how jaded I had become in the midst of all the attacks I had endured connected to my work on CTE.

"To come to California and become the county's new forensic pathologist. I work in this county as the director of the medical laboratory in the county hospital. They need a top-notch, highly competent pathologist like you to come in here and bring the whole operation up-to-date. Are you interested?"

Since I did not have a job and since I needed to find one quickly to avoid being deported back to Nigeria, I was indeed interested.

I called the captain back. He offered to fly Prema and me out to the San Francisco area for a five-day interview. This sounded like a vacation to me, so I accepted. When we arrived, we were treated like royalty. The difference between this and what we had endured over the previous few years was stark. Prema loved the place. She was ready to move right away. Me—I was hesitant. In California, the county coroner's office falls under the jurisdiction of the sheriff's department, placing police officers in charge of forensic autopsies. I had flashbacks to Nigeria, a corrupt country with a big government. The sheriff-coroner system is very out-of-date, as is the way in which the coroner is an elected office in most parts of America. The elected system seemed preferable to what I found in California. I was ready to turn the job down when Prema uttered five words that settled the question. "Bennet," she said, "I like it here." Then she added, "I want to raise my children here."

That settled it. We moved to Lodi, California, a community in the California wine country less than two hours from San Francisco, one hour from Napa Valley, and less than three hours from Lake Tahoe in the Sierra Nevada mountains. Coincidentally, I lived in Lodi, New Jersey, for a few months while doing my residency in New York. That particular Lodi did not work out, but this one was the perfect fit for the needs of my soon-to-be growing family.

I found peace in Lodi. The community did not revolve around a professional football team, like Pittsburgh does with regard to the Steelers. While San Francisco has an NFL team—and I imagine many people here are rabid fans—football culture did not permeate every aspect of social life in our new community. I needed that. A CTE research group in Boston had already started grabbing headlines. They had effectively pushed me out of the picture when it came to football and brain trauma. By this point, I was ready to oblige them. I was ready to settle into Lodi and get on with life. Eventually, we sold our house in Pittsburgh. Because we sold the house at the bottom of the housing market crash, we ended up losing close to a quarter of a million dollars on it. To me, this was one of the sacrificial costs of meeting Mike Webster. It was far less than the price he paid.

. . . .

In spite of my desire to remove myself from football and the NFL, I continued my brain research. In my new house in Lodi, I converted my garage into a brain tissue lab. Every morning, I woke up early, pulled the two cars out onto the driveway, turned on the floodlights, mounted my mobile table, and went to work. It was not work. Examining brains is something I truly enjoy. I guess I was born to be a neuropathologist. There in my garage, I examined the brains of a few famous athletes, but it was not about who they had been in life. I approached each individual with the same care, love, and reverence I show all of my patients. I did not conduct this research to make a name for myself, nor did I want to make headlines. This was a journey to find answers about CTE. I wanted to know how it spreads and why some people are more susceptible to it than others. While the Boston group grabbed more headlines, I was content to do my work in my garage. After all, many people have changed the world as they worked out of their garages. Because I did not have anyone funding my research, I had to support myself with whatever I had at my disposal. I continued to entrust Jonette Werley with processing the tissue samples, just as she had Mike Webster, Terry Long, Andre Waters, Justin Strzelczyk, Chris Benoit, Tom McHale, and every person whose brain I examined. She had the Midas touch. More than that, the way she works behind the scenes without recognition makes her my hero.

Between my new job and my continued research, I stayed very busy.

I also joined the faculty at the University of California, Davis, Department of Medical Pathology and Laboratory Medicine. Not a day went by that I did not read at least one scientific paper or textbook or professional article. My father preached that education empowers you to become anyone you want to be. I listened. Even after I stopped pursuing degrees, I continued pursuing an education, as I still do to this day and hope to do until I draw my last breath.

One morning, I awoke early, as was my habit. I sat down in my home office and looked out the window into the peaceful darkness and quiet of the night. I heard the sound of a car driving in front of my neighbor's house. The sound of the car was followed by the sound of a newspaper landing on his porch. I laughed a bit to myself at how old school my neighbor was that he still took the daily paper when out of the blue in the quiet of that moment, I heard a voice in my heart. *Bennet*, the voice said, *look at all the books you have read over the years.* I looked up at my bookshelf, which was loaded with books about everything from pathology, medicine, and public health to business and self-help. Then the voice in my heart said, *You have read all these books over the course of your lifetime, Bennet, but you have not read through the only book that should truly matter to you, the only book that should be closest to you as a child of the living God and a follower of Jesus Christ.*

Most people, at the sound of that voice, would have immediately pulled their Bible off the bookshelf and started reading. I could not do that because I did not have a Bible there to read. I had read bits and pieces of the Bible over the years, and I had heard it expounded upon in church all my life. Men like Father Carmen poured the Bible into me as they invested their lives into mine. But I did not have a Bible in my home to call my own. Just writing this right now leaves me embarrassed. How could I claim to be a Christ follower and not even own a copy of His Word?

I sat down at my computer and logged onto the Internet. Instead of checking my email, as was my habit, I Googled an online Christian bookstore and ordered a copy of the New American Bible. I clicked "overnight" on the delivery options. This was not my first time to purchase a Bible. I had bought Bibles before for myself and to give to others, but at that moment in my life, I had no Bible I could call my own. I had given away my last Bible several years prior to an addict I tried to help get off drugs.

After ordering the Bible, I tried to get to work, but I could not. I was too disappointed in myself to devote the rest of the morning to the pursuits I had chased while leaving God on the periphery. During my times of trouble, I had poured out my heart to Him and clung to Him by faith. He never let me down, but now I felt like I had let Him down. Terribly. I was so depressed that I went back to bed and back to sleep. I did not accomplish anything that day. The Bible I had ordered could not get to my house fast enough.

This was a turning point for me. Since that day, I have spent time every morning reading the Bible. It enlivens my spirit and invigorates and empowers my life. Over the previous years, I had fought so many battles in the world. Until I devoted myself to reading the Bible, I never realized how ill equipped I had been for those fights. More than that, spending time in the Bible keeps me from being immersed in and consumed by the affairs of this world. I believe I can see and understand the world system marked by conformational intelligence much better when my mind is shaped by God's Word. I have become mindful that I cannot let the conformations of society, the ways of the world, the earthly affairs of my life, or my daily burdens and worries eat up, scorch, or choke the word of God in me.[1] As Saint Paul instructed the Romans, "Do not conform yourself to this age but be transformed by the renewal of your mind, that you may discern what is the will of God, what is good and pleasing and perfect."[2]

• • • •

I needed the daily transformation and encouragement the Bible gave me because the marginalization that began with the publication of my first paper kicked into high gear in 2007 and 2008. I was surprised and appalled when my attention was drawn to a trend in the *New York Times* where the newspaper appeared to be joining the NFL to dehumanize me. When I reviewed the *Times* articles on CTE, a trend seemed obvious. In 2007, I was recognized for discovering CTE in several articles, but then as time went on, my name was systematically eliminated and never mentioned in their historical narrative of CTE. As more articles were published in the paper, other American doctors began to be recognized and even given the credit for discovering CTE. The name Omalu disappeared from the narrative in the most influential newspaper in America. Why such a respected paper would perpetuate a lie in such an un-American way baffled me. Was it because I was an immigrant, or I was black? I really do not know.

The *New York Times* was only the beginning. I wrote a third paper, one that focused on my discovery of CTE in the brain of Andre Waters. I started on this paper before leaving Pittsburgh. Even before I finished the paper, I had more and more cases come to me—from Justin Strzelczyk, Chris Benoit, and Tom McHale to Gerald Small, Altie Taylor, and others. I even discovered CTE in military veterans who had been diagnosed with PTSD and died from drug overdoses and suicide. However, I chose to focus the third paper solely upon Andre Waters, just as I had focused upon Mike Webster and Terry Long in the first two papers.

Once I finished the paper and went through the usual round of edits with my coauthors, I submitted it to *Neurosurgery* once again. Initially, the editors accepted the paper and started the review process that had by now become very familiar to me. The editors, reviewers, and I went back and forth with all the usual steps that must be taken before a paper is published. I reviewed references, corrected some editorial issues, and fixed all the typographical errors. The paper was nearly ready for publication when, like a thief in the night, Dr. Michael Apuzzo called and said, "I've changed my mind." When I asked why, he offered no explanation.

For years, I could only guess as to why this had happened. After all, there was nothing new in the third paper—no new, groundbreaking revelations. I had done that with the first paper. The third reinforced what I had written before. No longer was CTE an abstract scientific proposition. Three cases mark a trend, to say nothing of the many more cases I had to back it up beyond the first three.

I believe the editor may have been pressured to reject that paper, and I believe I know who may have pressured him. By 2008, when this rejection took place, it seemed that one or several journals of medicine had become the marketing and positioning pitch of the National Football League. There is a line in the movie *Concussion* that sums this up perfectly: "The NFL now owns neuroscience. Who knew?" At the time my third paper was rejected, *Neurosurgery* published a paper by the NFL research team concluding that NFL players are at lower risk of concussions because they have such strong necks.[3] This was followed by a study concluding that new and emerging helmet models could reduce the risk of serious concussions to such a degree that NFL concussions will rarely, if ever, transition to more serious brain injury.[4] They reached this conclusion by studying rats, not football players.

After *Neurosurgery* rejected my third paper, I sent it to other scientific journals. All turned me down as well. By now the word was out: I was dangerous, and my research should not be trusted. The rejections drove me to my knees in prayer. As the old saying goes, when a door closes in your face, God must have opened a window for you somewhere. My window had to lie outside of the establishment network of medical journals. My thoughts turned to a smaller journal for which I had done some work as a reviewer in the past. I contacted the editor and asked her if she would consider publishing my third paper. She agreed to take a look. After reading it, she had one question: Why did anyone pass on this?

A short time later, "Chronic Traumatic Encephalopathy in a National League Football Player: Case Report and Emerging Medico-Legal Practice Questions" appeared in the *Journal of Forensic Nursing*.[5] Since I had changed publications, I removed Part 3 from the title. I also presented Mike Webster's and Terry Long's cases and compared them to that of Andre Waters. The paper explored emerging symptoms they all shared—symptoms I thought were the defining signs of CTE. The paper came out in early 2010. To me, the truth had prevailed.

Or had it? After the third paper was rejected by *Neurosurgery*, one of my potential coauthors for that paper called me. "Bennet, I don't know what has happened to you since you moved to California. Your first two papers were sound, but this one is a mess." I dropped him as a coauthor. I later discovered he had close ties to the NFL. Another potential co-author, whom I had also dropped, later went on national television and questioned my competence, even though this individual held a PhD, not a medical degree. Some of my African-American friends who saw the interview called later and were very angry about some of the language he had used. I wondered how a person who was not a medical doctor could determine the competence of a medical doctor. I later discovered he had become an NFL consultant.

• • • •

I had begun to despair that the history of CTE, which was already in the process of being rewritten, would soon exclude me completely. The danger is that those who rewrote the history could also rewrite the truth that lies beneath it. I discovered CTE in an American football player only because I was an outsider whose thinking about that sport—and all contact sports—did not conform to the accepted ideas within the culture of this country. Because of this, my eyes looked for what others had not.

And what I could see is that football is not safe for the brain, and it *cannot* be made safe for the brain. Period. Others will tell you that we can make football safer with the right precautions and with new concussion protocols. Saying we can make football safer is no different from saying we can make a safer cigarette. Both statements are equally absurd, but when the public hears an expert say the league is taking steps to make football safer, their fears are alleviated. Everyone can then tune out the crazy Nigerian and keep watching and playing like usual. The one rewriting the history of CTE can then claim that "yes, the game caused harm to players in the past, but that is all in the past." There is nothing to worry about today, even though nothing has changed with the game. The dangers are not just in the past, but they are in the present and the future. I knew all of this was at stake, but there was nothing I could do to stop it. I presented myself to God and asked Him to guide me in defense of the truth. *Let Your truth prevail*, I prayed. Thankfully, God heard me.

In 2009, a brilliant and kind journalist named Jeanne Marie Laskas called me. She explained that she was doing a feature article for *GQ* magazine about football. As she began to research topics on which to focus, she discovered the growing crisis about brain trauma and CTE. Jeanne Marie went to Boston and interviewed many of the people who were now analyzing brains of deceased players for signs of the disease. In her research, she had discovered my story of how I discovered CTE in Mike Webster's brain. When she brought up my name, she heard things like, "His role is overblown," "Omalu is not to be trusted," and "He's not doing this kind of work anymore. We don't know where he is now or what he is doing."

The people she interviewed did not know where I was, but she decided to find me and discover the truth about me for herself. The result was a beautiful article called "Bennet Omalu, Concussions and the NFL: How One Doctor Changed Football Forever."[6] For the first time my story was told. At the time Jeanne Marie wrote the article, I had discovered eleven cases of CTE. The NFL and those connected to it might continue to dismiss me, but the truth had now been told. The fact that the truth is plain for all to see does not mean others will not continue to try to deny it. But I did not have to try to defend myself any longer. The truth had been told. The truth will defend itself.

But God was not finished answering my prayers for Him to defend the truth. Not long after the *GQ* article ran, my phone rang. I do not typically answer my phone when I do not recognize the number, but on this day, I noticed the call came from outside the United States. My curiosity was piqued. I took the call.

The man on the other end was very excited that I answered. He could barely get the words out as he said, "I am lying on the beach in Australia, and I just read the article about you. Why hasn't Hollywood turned your story into a movie?"

I almost laughed at the thought. *Why would Hollywood want to make a movie about me?*

Chapter Twenty-One

Omalu Goes Hollywood

For a story to go from magazine article to feature film takes more than a call from someone who knows someone in Hollywood. After the call from the man on the Australian beach, I started to wonder if my story of how I discovered CTE could really be adapted into a movie. I called Jeanne Marie Laskas, who had written the *GQ* article, and asked what she thought of the idea. Like me, she loved it, but she cautioned me to be careful with whomever I would be entrusting the film rights to my life. She introduced me to a man named David Wolthoff. David proved to be another angel sent by God into my life. Over the next few years, we walked together down a very long, arduous, and convoluted road that reminded me, once more, that God works all things out in the fullness of His time.

After a long conversation with David, I signed over the rights to my life story to him, and he started shopping it immediately. David had many meetings with studio after studio. Nothing came of it until Oprah Winfrey's Harpo Studios showed interest. I drove down to Los Angeles for a meeting with a couple of Harpo executives, which went really well. A short time later, they bought the options. My excitement dwindled as nothing happened for a long while. I kept doing my job, and David kept after Harpo to move forward. Eventually, they approached Peter Landesman, a journalist-turned-screenwriter, about possibly writing a script. He flew out to California to meet me. The two of us spent a day together. He also visited my home and met my family. After Peter's visit, my hopes were high. I thought we were on the cusp of the film becoming a reality—and then . . . nothing. As I was beginning to learn, there are a world of obstacles that must be overcome to go from story idea to feature film.

A couple more years passed. David kept aggressively pushing my story to anyone and everyone in Hollywood who would listen to him. Every now and then, he sent me an email or called to reassure me he had not given up. I continued doing research into CTE and brain trauma in my garage laboratory, while also teaming up with Dr. Julian Bailes, Bob Fitzsimmons, and another colleague and friend of mine, Jennifer Hammers, on joint efforts. I followed up the publication of my third paper with a fourth, titled "Chronic Traumatic Encephalopathy in a Professional American Wrestler," namely, Chris Benoit. Like the third paper, the fourth was also published in the *Journal of Forensic Nursing*.[1] I also wrote a paper exploring the link between CTE and suicide, which appeared in the *American Journal of Forensic Medicine and Pathology*.[2]

My next paper came out in 2011 in *Neurosurgical Focus*.[3] It focused on CTE in an Iraqi war veteran with Post-Traumatic Stress Disorder (PTSD) who had committed suicide. In 2010, I had discovered CTE in a sixty-one-year-old Vietnam War veteran who died suddenly. Because the symptoms of PTSD and CTE overlap in several areas, I wondered if much of what is diagnosed as PTSD in the military may have its roots in brain trauma. If not, I suspected the two might make each other worse. That is what led me to the case of a twenty-seven-year-old honorably discharged Marine who had suffered head trauma both while serving in Iraq and through recreational sports, specifically football and hockey. Prior to his death, he exhibited symptoms very much like those of the football players I had examined, including memory lapses, mood swings, extreme headaches with dizziness, and social withdrawal. My examination of his brain found the same telltale patterns of tau proteins across his brain: CTE.

That same year, 2011, I was back on the pages of *Neurosurgery* with a paper titled "Emerging Histomorphologic Phenotypes of Chronic Traumatic Encephalopathy in American Athletes."[4] *Neurosurgery* actually invited me, through Dr. Julian Bailes, to submit a new paper. I was shocked when Julian called with the news. However, my shock disappeared when he told me that Dr. Apuzzo was no longer the editor. He had been replaced by Dr. Nelson Oyesiku, a fellow Nigerian. Nigeria may have a reputation as a corrupt country politically, but it produces lots of high achievers. I am very proud of my heritage.

In writing this paper, my coauthors and I transitioned from "football players" to "athletes," because those who participate in all contact sports—most especially high-impact, high-contact sports—are at risk of brain trauma and therefore CTE. This includes those who play football, ice hockey, wrestling, boxing, mixed martial arts, and rugby. Lacrosse and soccer players are also at risk, due to incidental contact and trauma, as well as headers. Applying our research to all athletes in contact sports widened the scope of our research while also letting me talk about more than football. To be honest, by this point I had grown weary of football and the NFL. I compared my findings in the eleven cases of CTE diagnosis. After I submitted the paper, I was asked to remove a handful of statements and paragraphs. Reviewers complained about some of my methods, contending that they deviated from the norm in CTE research. I found it odd that a "norm" had emerged in such a new field, one that did not exist before September 2002.

Definitive diagnosis of CTE can only be done postmortem, while only presumptive diagnosis can be done in the living. Presumptive diagnoses are based on symptoms. After death, it is too late, as every family member I've ever had to tell that their loved one suffered from CTE has told me. This problem became very personal one day when I received a call from Tia McNeill.

Tia contacted me because she did not know where else to turn. Her husband, Fred, had played twelve seasons in the National Football League. After his career ended, he went to law school, graduated, and passed the bar. Tia and Fred had two sons. Life was good. But then

Fred began to forget things. He had trouble concentrating. Then came the headaches. He could not focus or stay on task, to such a degree that he lost his partnership at the law firm where he worked. Gradually his personality began to change. The easygoing, calm family man blew up at his kids and exhibited bouts of anger. He began making poor decisions, which resulted in money problems. The McNeills went bankrupt, losing their house. They separated not long after.

Listening to Tia pour out her heart to me, I felt sick to my stomach for her. I had heard variations of her story too many times and it always ended the same way. During her conversation, I finished sentences for her as she described Fred's symptoms. Tia was amazed. "Wow, how did you know?" she said over and over. I knew because of Mike Webster's family's stories and Terry Long's family's stories—and on and on and on.

A half hour after Tia called, she finally paused and said, "What do you think, Dr. Omalu?"

I told her the truth. "You know what? I would bet my life that your husband has CTE."

"What can we do to help him?" she asked.

That is the most difficult question anyone can ask me, because, honestly, there is nothing anyone can do to fix this problem. That is why we must find a cure. And the first step toward finding a cure is to be able to diagnose the disease definitively in a living patient beyond doing so symptomatically.

Like I have always done in my life, I do what I can as a person, in spite of what society thinks or what others think. Through the leadership of Julian Bailes and Bob Fitzsimmons, we identified a radiological marker for tau and amyloid proteins called FDDNP that was discovered at the University of California, Los Angeles. We formed a corporation called Taumark in order to purchase the intellectual property license on FDDNP so that no other group—the NFL, for instance—could purchase it and tuck it away. With the control we have on the intellectual property, Taumark raised money and carried out radiological scans of the brains of five retired NFL players, including Fred McNeill. The tests experimentally identified

CTE in their brains. Since then, we have scanned many more athletes and military veterans and actually discovered the "blast-variant" form of CTE in military veterans diagnosed with PTSD.

A couple of years after administering the Taumark test on Fred McNeill, he passed away. I performed the autopsy on his brain and confirmed the FDDNP findings. Not only did CTE shorten his life, but it also robbed him and his family of his true self over the last twenty years of his life. His would be the very first time CTE was identified in the brain of a living patient and confirmed when he died. That does not mean the issue of definitive diagnosis in the living has been solved by Taumark. Many years of expensive tests and clinical trials still lie before us before FDDNP may be approved by the FDA as a probable diagnostic tool for CTE and other dementias like Alzheimer's disease.

• • • •

Working with the McNeills gave me hope that I was making a difference. That hope was dashed not long after. When Junior Seau, yet another great retired NFL player, committed suicide in 2012, I was invited to assist with the autopsy. I removed his brain and spinal cord from his body and processed, prepared, and packaged them for analysis and transport with me on the plane. As I was about to leave for the airport, Junior Seau's son called the medical examiner's office and called me all types of names no man deserves to be called. He said I should not get anywhere close to his father's body. This was the same person who had given me verbal consent the previous night to examine his father's brain. Apparently some people had misinformed him about Bennet Omalu and fed him lies. Junior Seau's brain was taken from me and sent to the NIH. NIH doctors analyzed the brain and sent histologic sections of the brain across the country to a panel of neuropathologists to confirm what I believed: Junior Seau suffered from CTE. It should surprise no one that the NIH did not include me on the panel of neuropathologists who conducted the tests. What did I do wrong?

. . . .

As all of this went on, David Wolthoff continued shopping my story around Hollywood. One day, he took it to a beautiful Moroccan-American woman named Amal Baggar. She shared it with her boss, Giannina Scott, and Giannina showed it to her husband, Ridley Scott. The two of them had just watched the brilliant PBS documentary on the discovery of CTE, *League of Denial: The NFL's Concussion Crisis*, by Mark Fainaru-Wada and Steve Fainaru. Both the documentary and the book by the same name do a wonderful job of exposing the ways in which the NFL went to any lengths necessary to cover up the truth about brain trauma and football. The filmmakers interviewed me several times for the project, and part of my story is told in the book and documentary.

I believe the Holy Spirit touched Ridley Scott, together with his wife, through the documentary. They reached out to David, and by God's grace, Harpo Studios released its option and the Scotts took possession of it. They took the story to Sony Pictures, and the studio was immediately on board. All of a sudden, we had a deal. After waiting years for something to happen, we were in business in a matter of weeks after the Scotts came on board.

As God would have it, Ridley and Giannina reached out to Peter Landesman to write a script. They had no idea that Harpo Studios had approached him several years earlier. Some might call this a coincidence; I called it the handiwork of God. Peter later told me that when Ridley called him, he asked, "Do you know about Bennet Omalu?"

Peter laughed. "What do you mean do I know about him? I know him extremely well. I've been in his home and spent time with his family." I guess that sealed it. Peter was the man for the job of writing the script. God answered my prayers and put everything in place in His perfect timing. To me, the movie was simply a miracle.

When work began on the script, Peter invited me to come down to Hollywood to meet with him for a few days at Ridley Scott's production company, Scott Free. For three straight days, I sat in a conference room with a team that included Peter, Jeanne Marie Laskas, Amal Baggar, and David Wolthoff as I poured out every detail of my life's story. We started as early as 7:00 a.m. and went as late at 10:00 p.m. Everyone in the room asked me deeply penetrating questions about why I did what I did. I soon realized I no longer had any secrets. My whole life was about to become public knowledge, but I did not care, if in sharing my story, even one person might be helped.

Over those three days, I shared things I had never told anyone before. Peter Landesman took copious notes and recorded every session. Ridley and Giannina were abroad producing the films *The Martian* and *Exodus: Gods and Kings*, but they joined us by phone several times. My medical training kicked in through the process, and I began to detach myself from the entire experience. I did not want to be consumed by the intoxicating allure of it all. I chose not to make this about me. Yes, this was my story, but this movie needed to be about the journey and the people I encountered along the way, celebrating our common humanity.

On the last day, I was given the names of the three actors who were under consideration to play me. Denzel Washington, Idris Alba, and Will Smith. To say I was flattered by the options is an understatement. Denzel Washington's and Will Smith's bodies of work speak for themselves, while Idris Alba had already played the part of one of my heroes, Nelson Mandela. I kept quiet as those in the room discussed who would make the best choice. After much discussion, the consensus was that Will Smith was a better fit for my upbeat yet intense and complicated personality. Ridley Scott reached out to him once the script was finished. Though Will was involved in another movie at the time, he asked for the script. This too was the hand of God. Peter sent it to him.

Several days later, I was driving home from work after a very long day of testifying in court. The defense attorney attacked me, trying to cast doubt on the testimony I had given on behalf of the prosecution. By the end of it, all I wanted to do was get home to my family and put work behind me. During the drive, my phone rang. I looked at the caller ID and saw it was Peter Landesman. My heart jumped. I picked up the phone and yelled, "Peter! What's up? How are you doing, my friend?" I don't know why I was yelling, except that I could not control my emotions. I knew he was calling about the movie.

Peter replied in a very calm voice, "Bennet, calm down. I was just at Will Smith's house, and everything looks good."

"Are you kidding me? Wow!" I said. "You mean he might actually take the part?"

"He's thinking about it," Peter replied. "There's just one thing. He wants to meet you first."

"Oooohhhhhh. Really? Why? When?"

Peter ignored the why and went straight to the when. "Are you available tomorrow or Friday?"

"Yes. Either one. Anything for you, Peter," I said.

"Okay. Stand by. I'll let you know which is going to work for Will."

When I got home, I could hardly get the words out to Prema—I was so excited. Two days later, on Friday morning, the call came. A limo was going to pick me up at four o'clock and drive me to Sacramento for a flight to Los Angeles. I went to work but didn't accomplish much. Around two o'clock that afternoon, I went home and took a shower. I put on a blue suit and a starched white shirt. Prema walked into the bedroom, took a look at me, and said, "I don't think so. Bennet, that doesn't look right." She went over to my closet and picked out a light brown suit and a beige shirt with brown oxford shoes. After I changed, Prema stood back and looked me over. "That's much better." Out on the street I heard the limo pull up. Prema hugged me tight and whispered in my ear, "Good luck." Our daughter and son, Ashly and Mark, gazed in utter amazement and delight, not really knowing what was going on. I only told them that Daddy was going to work like I always did when I traveled to testify in court cases across the country.

I was nervous when I got into the limo. My heart was racing. Deep inside, I kept hearing the Spirit remind me, "Bennet, remember in medical school where you just wanted to be yourself? Now is the time. Be yourself. Just be yourself." I took a deep breath and settled into the seat.

"Be yourself." I ended up nodding off to sleep. An hour later, the driver woke me up and told me we were at the airport.

The flight from Sacramento to Los Angeles International Airport does not take long. Sony Pictures had booked me a first-class seat. I was not used to such luxury. After we landed at LAX, the same airport where I had landed when I first arrived in America so many years before, another limo driver greeted me. This was quite a change from 1994, when I wandered around the airport lost, looking for a toilet. Now I felt like the guest of honor. I climbed in the back of the limo, and we took off to where I did not know. After crawling along the freeways and streets of LA, the limo pulled up to the Bel Air Hotel. Bel Air was one of the most beautiful places I had ever seen. The cars coming and going at the hotel made my jaw drop. Movie stars mingled about.

Once inside the hotel, I did not know what to do. Thankfully, I heard someone call out, "Bennet." I turned to see Peter Landesman walking toward me. When we got close enough to talk, he looked me in the eye and asked, "Are you okay?"

"Yes, I am fine," I lied. Inside I was a nervous wreck. *Where am I? Why am I here? I do not belong here!*

Peter sensed what I was thinking. "Relax, Bennet. Right now you belong in this place as much as anyone else. Just mind your business, and do not let this place get to you. If you see a famous person, simply pretend you do not know them. They do not want you to go over and acknowledge them. That's not what they are here for, and neither are you. Okay?"

I swallowed hard. "Okay."

"Do you need a drink to calm you down?" Peter asked.

"Yes, very much," I said.

"So do I," he replied. He held my shoulders while leading me into the bar. Just as he had told me, famous people were everywhere. I did my best to ignore them. When we got to the bar, we heard a voice calling out, "Peter!" It was Giannina Scott, who had just arrived at the hotel and was walking to the bar to meet us. What a gorgeous, elegant woman, yet she too seemed a bit anxious. The three of us sat down at a table and ordered something to drink.

Peter, Giannina, and I sat and talked. Peter's assistant had told him that Will Smith was on his way. My heart began to race when he said this. From the moment Peter told me I was going to meet Will Smith, I had rehearsed in my mind what I was going to say to him. I did not want to come across as an overeager fan. No, I needed to be confident and comfortable. I planned on standing erect, face held high, and extending my hand and saying "Hi, Will. I'm Bennet." I rehearsed the line in my mind over and over.

About ten minutes after we arrived, a restaurant employee came over to inform us that Mr. Smith was waiting for us in a private dining room. I have to say that it is a very unusual experience to meet someone face-to-face whom you have only previously seen on a television or movie screen. Will stood as we walked over to the table. He walked over to Peter first and hugged him, and then he hugged Giannina. Because I am a short man, he could not see me behind them. "Where's Dr. Omalu?" Will asked.

Peter and Giannina stepped aside and stretched out their arms to introduce me. "Hi, I'm Will Smith," Will said, extending his hand.

As I shook his hand, I said, "I am Bennet Omalu. Please call me Bennet."

"And call me Will," he said.

"I am so honored to meet you," I said. My heart raced inside me. In my heart, I recited the prayer I had prayed so often since I came to America: *Jesus, I love You. All I have is Thine. Yours I am, and Yours I want to be. Do with me what Thou wilt.*

"It's an honor for me too," Will said. "Here, Bennet, sit next to me." He pulled his chair close to me, rested his forearm across the back of my chair, and engaged me in conversation. We hit it off right from the start. Our dinner began at about 7:30 p.m. At midnight, we were still talking.

One of the first questions Will asked me was, "Bennet, why do you do what you do? I've read about how much you've gone through. Why don't you stop? What can possibly be in this for you?"

"Growing up in Nigeria," I said, "the system was corrupt, and the people suffered from it. I dreamed of coming to America. When I was a boy, I believed America was heaven on earth, that this country was the closest to what God wants us to be as His sons and daughters. This was a country where you can be whatever you want to be, a country that gives you the platform to be yourself. I had this idealistic view of America, where I believed it was a place where there was no corruption, and the individual was the centerpiece that held the society together.

"When I discovered CTE in Mike Webster, I believed my discovery would be celebrated and embraced as a way of protecting those who were being harmed by football. But that did not happen. I experienced firsthand the way the NFL and the larger society degrade the individual and use them for their own purposes. The truth was being smeared, blurred, and covered up. So I rose up in anger to stand by the truth, not as a moralist, but as a child of God, as a man striving to find himself and live a life invested in the truth and the light of God in America, a land where there was, in my mind, no corruption."

Throughout the night, I poured out my heart to Will. A little after midnight, his phone rang. He then said, "I have to go." We said our good-byes and took a photo together. I rode in a limo to my hotel in Beverly Hills. I could hardly sleep after a night like that. Finally I managed to drift off.

At about 6:00 a.m. the next morning, my phone rang. "Bennet, you did it, man!" Peter shouted into the phone.

"What?" I said, trying to wake up.

"Will just called me. He's in. You know, he didn't want to do this picture. He's a big football fan, and he got what this movie is all about. His son played football. But after spending time with you last night, man, he's in. Now get your butt outta bed, and let's go celebrate!"

After I hung up the phone, all I could think was that God is good. I knew my story was in the best of hands. More than that, I knew the truth had prevailed.

Chapter Twenty-Two

Concussion

D r. Omalu, do you have a medical degree?" a voice asked.

"Yes, from the University of Nigeria at Enugu, Nigeria" came the answer—but not from me. An uncomfortable chill ran up my spine as I heard these words echo through the darkened theatre for the first time. The final edits to the movie had not yet been made, but for all intents and purposes, it was finished and playing on a big screen for me right then. The producers were anxious to get my reaction to the film. It was very important to them that I liked it. That was the reason behind this screening. Gugu Mbatha-Raw, the beautiful actress who so eloquently portrayed Prema, sat behind me. Other members of the cast and crew were scattered about the theatre.

When the lights went down and the movie began to play, the experience felt like watching any other movie. The film opens with Mike Webster's Hall of Fame speech. I had never heard it, and I found it fascinating. Then Will Smith appeared on the screen. He sat in the witness stand in a courtroom. The defense attorney addressed him as Dr. Omalu. Suddenly my moviegoing experience turned upside down. This was not at all like watching a movie. My brain could not process what this was. I had never experienced anything like it before. As a physician, I knew what was happening to me. I was in shock. *How is it possible that my life is on this movie screen?* my mind screamed at me.

I know that last sentence is difficult to believe. In my head, I knew a movie was being made about my life. I had spent a great deal of time with the writers and with Will Smith and had served as a technical consultant for the crew as they tried to get all the details just right. Some days my email in-box filled up with nearly a hundred questions regarding the movie. My phone rang constantly as I answered question after question. I even spent time on the set and flew back to Pittsburgh, as parts of the movie were filmed there. Cyril Wecht and I reconnected through the making of this movie. So if you had asked me, "Bennet, do you know they are making a movie about your life starring Will Smith as you?" I would have said to you, "Of course I know. What a stupid question!"

However, when I sat down in the theatre and watched the film for the very first time, I found I was totally unprepared for the mental conflict in my mind. As Will Smith answered the defense attorney's questions in a strong and accurate Nigerian accent, my head began to spin. I fell into a somewhat trancelike state. My brain could not process the information that my eyes and ears sent it. People on the screen were talking to me, and I was answering, but it was not me. Slowly I began to realize that I was watching a movie about myself. I know that sounds like a very silly statement, since I had aided in the making of the very movie I was now watching. Yet there is a big difference between knowing and experiencing. My mind struggled to accept the experience.

I remained in this state until the midpoint of the movie—trying to watch and trying not to watch at the same time. Shock gave way to a wave of positive emotions in the scene where Will Smith (as me) asked Prema to marry him. When I heard Gugu (as Prema) say, "If you want to marry me, I will marry you," a flood of memories rushed over me. Tears welled up in my eyes. More wonderful memories came. The tears began running down my face in rivulets. Thankfully, I was prepared, for I had a handkerchief with me. I was also thankful the theatre was dark; I don't think anyone noticed me crying.

The tears kept coming until the movie came to an end. When the final scene was over, I sat and stared at the screen. I did not even know the theatre lights had been turned up. Gugu left the theatre. I did not notice.

Concussion

Finally I gathered myself and stood up. I turned and faced the producers and crew and everyone else connected with the film who sat behind me. No one said a word. Then I smiled and gave a thumbs-up. The theatre broke out in applause and cheering. The editorial team seemed the most exhilarated. Peter Landesman came over to me. "How was it?" he asked. He wanted more than a thumbs-up response.

"Most beautiful. I love it. Thank you so much, Peter, and may God bless you," I replied.

Peter hugged me. "I'm glad you like it," he said.

I left the theatre, but my legs had trouble carrying me. The experience of seeing all I had gone through over the previous thirteen years play out on screen overwhelmed me. I felt numb. It was more than the impact of the movie itself. Watching the film released all of the emotions I had experienced since the day I met Mike Webster and began searching for answers for him. Through the movie, those answers would soon be on display for all the world to see. The truth was going to prevail. No doubt some could still deny the truth, but their voices would ring hollow.

When I arrived at my hotel, I went up to my room and went straight to bed, I did not stir for twelve hours.

The next time I watched the movie, I had a different experience. Unlike the first screening, the second time I watched the film I was able to sit back and take it all in. I must say, watching Will Smith on the screen was like watching a taller—and my wife would say better-looking—version of myself. I forgot I was watching Will Smith. He became me.

The transformation became most apparent to me in the first scene, where Will performs an autopsy. The moment made me smile. In preparation for the role, Will and Peter came to Lodi to watch me work. The two of them stood beside me during an autopsy. I made sure there were chairs in the room where they could sit down when the sights, sounds, and smells became too much. Will was a good student, for when he performed an autopsy on the screen, I saw my own mannerisms and heard myself saying the very things I say to my patients as I work on them. During the many hours Will and I spent together as he prepared for the role, he once said to me, "Bennet, do not worry. I will do you justice." He was true to his word.

The second time through, I was also able to appreciate some of the smaller touches Peter Landesman and Ridley Scott made sure to include. In an early scene where Will is driving along in his Mercedes, the image of a jetliner is reflected in the car windshield. For most people, this meant nothing. To me, I knew this was an acknowledgment of how I had never wanted to be a doctor; I had wanted to be an airline pilot.

Another image made me choke up with emotion, and it does every time I watch the movie. Several times in the film, the camera shows a photograph on the wall. In one scene, Gugu asks Will, "Is this your father?" The photograph was indeed a photograph of my father. Will first saw the picture on a visit to our home in Lodi. He asked me that same question. I told him my father's story, which touched him. Unfortunately, my father did not get to see the movie. He died in May 2014 at the age of ninety-one during the early phases of the film's production. I still cannot believe he is gone. When I shared this story with Will, he said to me, "We must include your father in this film to honor him." The appearance of his photograph in the movie was all because of Will.

The movie went through a few more revisions and final edits after the initial screenings I watched at the Sony studios. When everything wrapped up, I went back home to Lodi and tried to resume my normal work routines. However, Sony kept me busy on projects related to the film. I was gone more than I was home, which I did not like. I hated being gone from my family, but I knew this was only temporary. Besides, I knew Sony had something special in store for all of us.

• • • •

It was a not-so-cold early November night in Los Angeles. I found myself in the backseat of a black Cadillac Escalade. Prema sat opposite me. Behind us our daughter, Ashly, and son, Mark, chattered away in somewhat reserved excitement about what was to come. The chauffeur picked us up at the Four Seasons Hotel in Beverly Hills, one of the nicest hotels I have ever stayed in. The only hotel to which I can compare it is the Burj Al Arab Hotel in Dubai where my family stayed in the summer of 2012 during the first vacation I had ever taken since coming to the United States. We took that trip to celebrate Prema's obtaining her U.S. citizenship. This ride in the back of the black Escalade through the streets of Los Angeles was another celebratory trip.

As we rode along in the back of the car, my family looked and felt like the great American success story I had always aspired to become—someone I used to see only in magazines and movies. I wore a beautiful, custom-made black suit; a crisp, custom-made white silk shirt; a blue-black tie; and black, executive shoes. My son wore a tuxedo and a big smile. Ashly looked beautiful in a formal blue-black dress with a white sweater. I tried to talk Prema into buying a long black evening dress for the occasion. She said no in no uncertain terms. "I prefer pants and a jacket," she told me while we shopped for our wardrobes for the night. I pressed the issue until the assistant who was helping us pulled me aside and told me to let my wife wear whatever made her feel comfortable. Prema ended up selecting gray Giorgio Armani pants and a matching jacket. She looked beautiful. I wondered why I ever questioned her judgment.

Prema was very quiet and meditative during the drive, while my kids talked so fast to each other in their adoptive American accents. I have never been able to develop the classic American way of talking, no matter how hard I try. My children speak so fast and so American that I sometimes cannot understand what they are saying. They only know a handful of words in my wife's and my native languages. They can ask, "Kedu?" which means "How are you?" in Igbo, and can say "Jambo bwana," which means "Hello, mister" in Prema's native Swahili.

"We're almost there, sir," the chauffeur said. Driving down the streets of Hollywood, I saw so many famous sights I had first seen in the movies growing up in Nigeria. I honestly did not know exactly where we were going. Sony personnel—so many of them young, beautiful women and young, handsome men—were essentially managing my life. They made air reservations for me, sending me to different parts of the country in the first-class cabins of commercial jets. Once or twice, I even flew in a private jet with Will Smith and his wife, Jada. Sony also put me in the best suites in the finest hotels across the United States. They took such good care of me, yet I was almost like a zombie, going where they told me to go when they told me to go there. Over the past few weeks, I had been so occupied with media appearances that in one city, one of the young women packed my clothes in my hotel room while I spoke with reporters in another part of town. Because I did not have time to get back to the hotel and check out before rushing off to the airport to catch another flight, she packed all my clothes, toiletries, medications, and even my underwear—something no one had ever done for me before, not even my wife.

"Here we are, sir," the chauffeur said as he pulled the Escalade up to the front of the world-famous TCL Chinese Theatre on Hollywood Boulevard. The place was glamour defined. So beautiful. So majestic. Any other time, my family and I might have walked around the grounds of the theatre and looked at the footprints in the concrete of so many Hollywood legends, but that was not possible tonight. Floodlights were everywhere. A red carpet extended out to the curb where we had parked. Ropes stretched out beside the red carpet, behind which stood so many excited and loud people who all looked happy to see us.

The chauffeur opened the car door. I climbed out as cameras flashed. I helped Prema out of the car. She looked nervous. My kids climbed out. Both had huge smiles on their faces, but I could tell they were also unsure of what was happening around them. This was a long way from our very private life in Lodi.

We lined up and prepared to walk up the red carpet. An announcer said, "Dr. Bennet Omalu and family." I put on a grin I had practiced for hours in front of a mirror at home. More cameras flashed around us. Television crews lined up and filmed our walk up the carpet. *Do not be afraid*, I heard the Lord say. I thought back to my father and the trip he took in the back of a car when he was about the age I was now. Then he had escaped with his life. Now his son and daughter-in-law and grand-children were being treated like royalty. I wondered if he heard the Lord whisper, *Do not be afraid*, as he made a long journey through war-torn Nigeria. Oh, how I wish he could have lived to see the movie and the vindication for the truth that it offered.

I took Prema by the hand and led her and the children to a Sony executive, who led them into the theatre while I stayed back on the red carpet to do interviews. Before we left Lodi, I told her what I experienced when I saw the movie for the first time. "This may be very emotional for you, because it was for me. It's okay. We will get through it," I said to her. Walking into the theatre for the world premiere of *Concussion*, I did not feel excited or expectant or any of the other emotions I thought I might feel. I was simply present in the moment.

Deep down, I knew that as soon as the movie hit the theatres, our lives were going to be disrupted for a time, something I did not need. Early on, a Sony consultant came to our house to brief me on what to expect from having a movie made about my life while I was still living. He told me that it is like winning the lottery. For some people, this is a good thing, but for many others, their lives end up in a bad place as a result of all the attention the movie brings. "Don't let it consume who you are," he told me. Will Smith said the same thing to me on one of the days we spent together. While showing him how to use a microscope, he looked over and said, "Bennet, this is who you are. Never give this up. Don't let the movie or anything else take your life away from you."

In the days and weeks leading up to the premiere, I reminded myself of their words. Now that the premiere was here I repeated a prayer reminiscent of the one the Virgin Mary prayed when Gabriel the angel told her she would give birth to the Christ.[1] I prayed, *Lord, may it be done to me according to Your word. I trust in You.* Then I prayed the prayer that has come to define my life: *Jesus, I love You. All I have is Thine. Yours I am, and Yours I want to be. Do with me what Thou wilt.* Out of the corner of my eye, I watched Prema. She remained very quiet. She hadn't asked for any of this, but she took it all in and did what needed to be done.

My children, on the other hand, soaked in every camera flash and all the glamour of the moment.

Once everyone was in the theatre, Peter Landesman introduced the movie. The theatre was packed, with people standing along the sides. In the middle of his introduction, Peter asked me to stand. I was not aware he was going to do this. When I stood, the applause thundered around me. People continued clapping for at least a minute. "Prema," I mouthed to my wife, "stand with me." She shook her head, NO. A quiet woman who does not like the limelight, she had had all she could stand. I did not press the issue. My children, however, stood up next to me. I think they enjoyed the moment. They felt very important.

The applause finally ended. Peter completed his introduction. The lights fell. The movie began. The audience was dead quiet when they should be silent, cried when they should cry, and laughed when they should laugh. Peter did a marvelous job of weaving together all the emotional elements in the film. Watching the movie with my family and a packed theatre full of people was a very different experience from watching it alone.

When the final credits rolled up on the screen, I thought this was the end. A premiere party was planned for later, and I looked forward to having some fun. A Sony executive came over and asked me to follow her to the greenroom. "Is it okay if my family comes too?" I asked. I knew Will was going to be back in the greenroom for a post-film talk by the producers. I knew my children wanted to see him again.

"Of course," the executive replied.

We went back to the greenroom, where I thought we would wait out the question-and-answer session going on upon the stage in the theatre. Once it was over, we would all go to the premiere party. However, to my surprise, once I was in the greenroom, someone came over to me and said, "Bennet, get ready."

"For what?" I asked.

"You are going on stage."

"On stage? Why?"

"For the panel discussion. Get ready."

A short time later, I found myself standing behind a black curtain, waiting. Then I heard my name called. The Sony executive opened the curtain, and I walked out on stage. The thunderous cheers, applause, yelling, and screaming took my breath away. The floodlights shining upon me blurred my vision. I looked over to the far side of the stage. Will, Peter, and the others on the panel were clapping and yelling as well. I got even more confused, almost to the point of fear. I began saying the same good old prayer: *Jesus, I love You. All I have is Thine. Yours I am, and Yours I want to be. Do with me what Thou wilt.*

I walked with trepidation across the stage, raised my hands, and began waving to the audience. I hugged Will and walked over to the empty chair and looked out at the theatre. Most people were still yelling and screaming. I could not make out people's faces because of the floodlights. I stood to Will Smith's left. He sat down, and I sat down. I was unsure what to do next. The moderator began speaking, and for the next hour, he led a Q&A session. Many people had questions for me. Answering them, I became another person—a person I did not even know. God has His sense of humor, and He manifests it in our lives and when we do not even expect it.

While I was on that stage, my mind wandered, and I asked myself, *Bennet, could this be you? Could this be you? Look at how far you have traveled from the war-torn village in Nigeria and air bombardments and malnutrition to a difficult childhood plagued by extremely low self-esteem. For so long, you struggled with who you are and battled depression. You thought these battles were behind you when you came to America, yet they followed you here. In America, you faced ever-increasing depression, cultural shock, and rejection in America as an outsider, as a black African man in mainstream America who had an accent and looked different. Look at how far you have come. By faith the impossible becomes possible.*

The impossible becomes possible, I said again and again to myself. The phrase has since become a part of every speech I deliver. My experience has shown me that all you have to do is to believe that, come what may, whatever will be will be—for God is on His throne. He is in charge.

All I must do is trust Him and entrust myself to Him. By faith in Him, the impossible becomes possible, no matter how small the faith may be: "Amen, I say to you, if you have faith the size of a mustard seed, you will say to this mountain, 'Move from here to there,' and it will move. Nothing will be impossible for you."[2] In fact, it was this night that I realized the mountain Jesus was talking about here was not the mountain in front of us, but the mountain inside of us. The biggest mountain we must overcome is the mountain of you, and the mountain of me. Remember, we are sons and daughters of a mighty God, the God who created the heavens, the universe, the earth. He created the sun and the moon and the mountains and the skies. He created me. He created you. And He breathed upon us His Spirit.

You and I are children of God, as majestic as the starry skies of night and as majestic as the sun. We are as illuminating as the sun. We are like the stars, the sun, the moon, the skies, the mountains, the universe. So if by faith I tell the mountain of me to move, it moves. Not because I am the one moving it, but because the God of the impossible makes all things possible in me. It may take a long time coming, but in the fullness of His time, it will come. Always dream the impossible dream, and by faith that impossible dream will become possible. Standing on the stage at the premiere of *Concussion*, I saw this impossible journey reach heights I never imagined possible. But it was not the end of the journey. No, in many ways it was just getting started.

Chapter Twenty-Three

From Doctor to Dad: What Will I Say When My Son Asks, "Can I Play Football, Pleeeaaaassse?"

My middle name, Ifeakandu, is an Igbo name that means "life is the greatest gift of all." I thought I understood the value of this gift through the life God has given me. Then, at the age of thirty-nine, I became a father for the first time. Holding my first child for the first time, I came to understand the real meaning of Ifeakandu. I knew this little girl, this life, is the greatest gift.

When Prema learned she was pregnant, neither of us took this gift of life for granted. But after losing our first child, we prayed anxiously for our second child's life. When Prema passed the point where we had lost our first baby, we both breathed a sigh of relief. When she reached full-term, we both grew anxious and excited. We had transformed part of our home into the baby's room. Now this little one just needed to come out into the world to enjoy it.

Prema's first contraction came while we were at home. We immediately started timing their frequency. Throughout most of the day, they remained very sporadic. Our baby had signaled she was ready to meet us face-to-face, but she was not in a hurry. Prema was actually in labor for almost two days. Finally the labor pains became stronger and more frequent. We rushed to the hospital. Our baby decided to take a little longer still. All throughout the night, we timed contractions. The time was growing closer. Eventually, Ashly arrived early in the morning. I remember her first noise, her first cry. It was miraculous and magical. I felt like heaven had come down to earth. Holding her for the first time, I could not believe this life had come from Prema and me. We had begotten life—the greatest gift of all.

After such a long labor and delivery, Prema was exhausted. We spent a good deal of time holding Ashly before the nurses came and took her so Prema could get some rest. I rushed home to take a shower and take care of a couple of things. I went back to the hospital as quickly as I could. By the time I returned, the nurses had cleaned up my baby girl for me. I took her in my arms. "Hello, cutie pie," I said. She opened her eyes at the sound of my voice and breathed in deep, like she was taking in the scent of her father. Those eyes looked up into mine. I felt like I was looking into the eyes of God. I became overwhelmed with emotion. Tears rolled down my face—tears of joy. I realized right then that in the process of conception between a man and a woman, God invites us to partake in His glory and share in His holiness and godliness. The creation of life is a holy experience. The baby girl I held close to my bosom was His gift of life.

Two years later, I enjoyed the same experience with the birth of our son, Mark. Being the bold boy that he is, Mark was in a hurry to come into the world. His labor was precipitous. We actually went to the hospital for an elective cesarean section birth, but Mark could not wait. I dropped off Prema and rushed out to take Ashly and our nanny back home. When I arrived back at the hospital less than twenty minutes later, Mark had already been born. As soon as I walked into the room, he heard my surprised voice and began crying loudly. The nurse handed my little boy to me. The moment he landed in my arms his crying stopped.

Again, when I felt Mark's warm body up close to my bosom, I felt like God was touching me. I had come from nowhere, with nothing—and now I had a son in my arms. Once again, I was overwhelmed with emotion. I cried and cried while my baby son slept in my arms. It was a tender moment I will never forget.

In the days after the births of Ashly and Mark, I felt a great burden to be a good father for them. God gave me the responsibility to lead and guide them and teach them about God and His creation. I am charged with teaching them about the great gift of life God has given them and show them how to make the most of this life. From the start, the two of them watched everything I did and said. They emulate everything I do. Many times they will ask me why I do what I do or say what I say. They ask me questions I never thought about before. Such are the joys and challenges of being a parent. These two precious lives ask me questions as they form their own unique personalities. They are growing up to be their own selves, the people they were born to be. After all, as parents we are only conduits and vessels of God's love. I do not own my children, and I cannot control the choices they make. But I can guide them—both by my words and by my example.

My words and my example and the words and example of my wife are not the only words and examples shaping my children's lives. They are surrounded by their peers and classmates. The two of them are immersed in a culture very different from the one in which I grew up in Nigeria or the one in which Prema grew up in Kenya. My children are becoming their own individuals, with Ashly's love of books and Mark's potent imagination, but they are also part of a larger community. And as part of that community, they will want to fit in and be like everyone else. Since a large part of the social context in America revolves around sports, my children will one day want to participate. I have written much about contact sports, but the question I face is very different when those precious eyes of my son or daughter look up at me as they ask, "Daddy, can I play football [or wrestle or take karate or join in one of the other very popular contact sports]?"

The question is difficult for every parent, even for me. I know how valuable sports are in the life of a child. Physical activity helps them develop into healthy adults, while playing on a team teaches them a great number of things about working together with other people and sacrificing oneself for the greater good. I want my children to play sports. I look forward to sitting in the stands and cheering them on as they strive to be the best they can be.

However, as a father, I will do my children a great disservice if I do not protect them from that which can cause them lifetime harm. I am not an overprotective parent. I do not try to keep my children from all risks. Prema and I did not cover the ground under our swing set with pillows and wrap our children in bubble wrap, lest one of them accidentally goes down the slide the wrong way. When I refuse to allow my children to play football or ice hockey or to do headers in soccer, I am not being overprotective; instead, I am protecting the great gift God has given them.

We do this as a society. When Prema and I brought Ashly and then Mark home from the hospital, we strapped them into car seats that appeared to have been designed by NASA engineers. The hospital where they each were born even offered a service to check to make sure the car seat was properly installed. Properly installed car seats for children is a very big issue in our country today, according to many parenting blogs. In most states, children must by law ride in some sort of protective seat until they are nine or ten years old. The reason is simple: as a society we value our children and want to protect them at all costs.

Yet it seems very odd to me that a parent will strap their child into a protective seat and then drive them to football practice, ice hockey practice, or rugby practice or allow that child to participate in mixed martial arts, boxing, or wrestling. Up until I discovered CTE, most parents assumed that the biggest risk their children faced when playing a high-impact, high-contact sport was a broken bone or perhaps some scrapes and bruises. We now know that those are the least of the dangers. Bones will mend, and scrapes will heal, but the damage done to the brain through concussive and subconcussive hits will last a lifetime.

My son, Mark, is almost seven years old at the time of this writing, but he already loves to use big words. Every now and then, he uses a new four- or five-syllable word on me, words like *gargantuan, duplication,* or *obtundation.* "Where did you learn such a big word?" I ask with wonder. He will just stare back at me with a look that says, *What are you talking about, Dad. These words aren't big. They are just my vocabulary.* I love to watch his intellectual curiosity grow. Why, then, would I take a chance on letting him play a game that might change his brain and make him incapable of fully realizing the gift of his mind that God has given him?

Some parents think I am overreacting. "We now have greater awareness about concussions," they say. "Coaches now teach the safe way to tackle on the football field or check another player in the hockey rink," they argue. These arguments do not hold water. Blows to the head are an integral part of games like football. You cannot take them out of the game. I know. I have watched football. During my research into CTE while writing my first paper, I watched high school teams practice. In those practices, young men lined up opposite each other and threw themselves into each other. The loud, clacking sound of plastic helmets hitting each other echoed across the field. Such was not an unusual sound. It is football.

"Your experience was a long time ago," some will say. "Over the past few years, football has changed. The game has become safe," they argue. This is the lie football leagues want you to believe. It is also a lie American culture is eager to believe. Football is more than a game; it is the centerpiece of many of our cultural events.

I know this from experience. I attended my first football game in the fall of 2013 at the invitation of a close friend. The two of us had been involved in a successful meeting, and all the participants were invited to attend the game at a nearby major college campus. The first thing I noticed when I arrived at the stadium was that this was not just a game. The pomp and pageantry of the event expressed the celebratory exuberance of America like nothing else can. I made my way to the VIP box reserved for our group. All of the conversations revolved around what was about to happen on the field. An excitement filled the air—a festival feeling that reminded me of the Brazilian carnival. The lights and the music and the seductive, undulating dances of the cheerleaders all fed the party atmosphere. I felt myself getting caught up in it.

The same mood permeated the VIP booth. Of course, alcohol and food flowed. This was a party no one wanted to miss. I found a seat and focused on the players on the field. I noticed most were young black men. They jumped around the sidelines with excitement. I knew these poor college kids believed they were doing something good. To be the center of attention at such an event had to be intoxicating for them. The young men all came to attention as the national anthem played and the flag was unfurled on the field. This was a truly American experience, where love for country and love for sport come together in one place.

Then the game started. The noises and sounds of the hits—head to head, helmet to helmet, body to body, head to body—they were simply unbearable for me. I could not believe that the sounds of the impacts were so loud, especially the crackling noises of helmet-on-helmet collisions. Early on, one player staggered after a hard hit and fell. He stayed down for about thirty seconds to a minute, stood up, and then ran about shaking his head and body with his upper extremities held out in a way that reminded me of a ritualistic dance to show he was potent and strong. I wondered how strong his brain was after that hit. Every human brain is equally vulnerable, whether you are a six-foot-six, 350-pound giant or a lovely four-year-old girl. This player showed how strong he was, even though his head was obviously foggy. I felt sick for him, while everyone around me was yelling and cheering on his aggressive play. Thank God I had to leave early to catch a flight back to California.

Unfortunately, before I left, I had to go down to the sidelines to meet and greet some people. The collision noises that seemed loud high up in the luxury box were now nearly deafening up close, and they surprised me by their sheer violence. I could not believe the brutality, and yet people cheered. During my few minutes on the sidelines, the microscopic images of the injured brains of all the players I had autopsied flashed through my mind. I was overwhelmed. My chest tightened, and

I found it difficult to breathe. I had to leave before I suffered a cardiac arrhythmia. The healer in me as a physician and the compassion in me as a Christian were repulsed by what I was experiencing. I had had enough. Standing there was mental and intellectual torture for me. You may call me a weakling of a man, and I freely accept that, for I am what I am. Yet strength does not mean watching young men, primarily young black men, inflict possible lifetime mental and psychological problems upon themselves for the sake of the entertainment of the thousands in the stands and the millions watching on television.

At what price are we to be entertained?

All of the young men who participated in the game I attended were over the age of eighteen. I would never restrict their right to choose to play this violent, brutal sport. However, as a father, when my underage child asks if he can play football, it is my duty as a father to say no. That does not mean I am saying no to sports. My children and my wife and I all watch the Olympic Games when they come around every four years. Those games are, to me as a dad, like taking my children through an endless buffet line. If they want to play a sport, the Olympics present them with so many choices of noncontact and less-contact sports. From track and field and swimming to volleyball and basketball; from badminton, lawn tennis, and table tennis to kayaking, rowing, and even cycling—the choices are all there. Do these sports draw the same crowds and garner the same passion from their fans as football in America? No, but does that matter? Sports are for those who play and enjoy them, not for the fans watching on the sidelines. As a father, I want to help my children find a sport they enjoy and one in which they can excel—and then to stand back and cheer them on. If no one else attends their game, so be it. These games are for my children's enjoyment, not to entertain others.

• • • •

To be honest, my children have not yet asked about playing football or other high-impact, high-contact sports. The questions I most often receive are like the one in the email I received early one Sunday morning. I got up that day later than I usually do, around 6:00 a.m. After reading my Bible and spending time in prayer, I made myself a cup of strong tea and went into my home office to review emails before my children woke up. At the top of my email in-box was a message from a name I did not recognize. In it, I found a long letter from a father and a leader in his community. He told me the story of his son, who was away at college—a son who was also a very successful football player. The dad described his son as a good boy from a good family who has had a very good life. The son's future looks promising, the father said, with the boy standing a very good chance of being drafted to play in the National Football League.

But there was more to the story.

The son had begun playing football in middle school and continued on through high school and now in college. A few years ago, the father began to notice changes in his son. The boy showed increasing impulsivity, anger control issues, and violent tendencies. Although all of these had never been present in his son's personality before, the dad dismissed them as the permissible excesses of a successful athlete. But over time, the symptoms became progressively worse. The boy, now a young man, became verbally and physically abusive at home. The dad also noticed subtle memory problems in his son. The dad passed off the memory issues as a sign of a very busy young man who had too much going on to remember every little detail.

Then the dad watched the movie *Concussion*. That was why he emailed me early on a Sunday morning. "I fear for my son," he wrote. "Could football have irreparably damaged his brain? What can I do to help him?" Yet this plea for help was followed by a reaffirmation of the son's bright future and his prospects of having a career in the NFL. This dad was very proud of his son and all that he had accomplished—proud, but also conflicted. He wanted his son to play professional football and enjoy the fame and money it might bring, but he also feared that if his boy continued to play, the damage to his brain might become even worse. "Please, Dr. Omalu, what should I do?" he asked.

I replied to his email right then. His son was not my son, and I had no say in what his son should or should not do. However, as a fellow father, I saw his son like my own. I told him that if this was my son, I would not let him play any longer. Even if damage has already been done, getting him off the football field will prevent more blows to the head and even more damage. We do not know exactly how many blows to the head will cause brain damage or which blow will be the one to make that damage irreversible and permanent. Since we do not know, the best thing this parent could do is to protect the future brain health of his son. If that means walking away from a possible career in football, so be it. When you consider the alternative, isn't it worth it?

I also advised this dad to encourage his son to engage in positive and healthy living. He should be careful about what he eats and drinks. If there is the possibility of brain damage already, he should avoid alcohol, which exacerbates the problems. I also told the dad to have his son take brain-friendly multivitamins and micronutrients like omega fatty acids. Finally, I advised him to take his son to see a neurologist in a university hospital that has a competent brain injury program. They should run a battery of tests to evaluate the level of any possible brain trauma and advise them on whatever steps are necessary for further treatment.

There's also one other piece of advice I give to dads like this one: forgive yourself. I have met parents and coaches who sob, some on my shoulders, who cannot get over what they "did" to their children or players. A youth football coach I know stopped coaching after he saw the movie *Concussion*. His two sons played football from the time they were big enough to strap on a helmet. Both sons today have serious memory, academic, mood, and behavioral problems. They are in their twenties. Their dad broke down as he began to talk to me about what life might be like for them in their thirties and beyond. "If I had only known," he said through his sobs.

But that is the point: *he did not know*. How could he have known? The truth of the inherent dangers of high-impact, high-contact sports to brain health had not been widely disseminated. Up until recent years, concussions were passed off as the mildest of brain injuries, as nothing to worry about. We know better now, and we should have known then. The truth was out there, but the truth was hidden and denied by those who had an interest in suppressing it. "You must forgive yourself," I told this father, "or else you will be so burdened by guilt that you cannot help your sons today."

As we now move forward as moms and dads and as children of the living God, it is foolhardy for any of us to ignore what we now know. I pray that the light of Christ may shine upon us, open our minds and hearts, and enlighten us in the path of truth. Let us protect, celebrate, and live our lives in the abundance of His truth and His love. Amen.

"I Bet My Medical License That O. J. Simpson Has CTE"

A round the time of the Golden Globe Awards, which I was privileged to attend with Will Smith, I did an interview with *People*
magazine. The journalist who interviewed me informed me that a new
television series about O. J. Simpson was going to premiere soon. He
asked if he could discuss the series with me. I said, "Sure." I then added,
without even giving it a thought, "I bet my medical license that O. J.
Simpson has CTE." Within a matter of hours, the interview was out, and
my phone began to ring. It did not stop ringing for days. I think every
journalist in America must have called, and those who didn't call must
have emailed me because my in-box filled up. Talk shows wanted to have
me on as a guest, and news shows wanted to do follow-up interviews—all
to discuss the case of O. J. Simpson. Many people accused me of defend-
ing O. J., as if I was saying he was not responsible for his murderous acts.
That was not my intention at all.

When I made the statement about O. J. Simpson, I made it on the
basis of scientific facts. Not many people know it, but in the United
States today, a large percentage of the prison population has a history of
traumatic brain injury. When a person is exposed to any type of traumatic brain injury, their risk of engaging in criminal activity increases.
Traumatic brain injuries increase one's disinhibition, making it more

difficult for persons to control themselves and their emotions, especially in stressful situations. It also increases one's risk of exhibiting exaggerated reactions and responses to daily life stressors and situations. In addition, brain trauma increases the risk of impairments to judgment and engaging in risky behavior, including sexual improprieties, to say nothing of the cognitive impairment and impaired executive functioning. This is not just my opinion; these are scientific facts.

My statement about O. J. and CTE is based on the facts I just cited. People have asked how O. J. could go from one of America's most beloved sports icons to an alleged murderer (although a court of law acquitted him of all charges). The same holds true of many current and former sports stars, especially football players. Every week, a story appears in a newspaper about a current or former player who committed domestic abuse or sexual assault or any number of other violent crimes. Many of these have had no history of violence. And people wag their heads and talk about these bad apples who have disgraced the programs for which they play.

I believe these are not all bad apples. I believe many are good men who have been changed as a result of brain trauma. The problem is that our culture does not want to admit that the games with which we are intoxicated could exact this toll on those who play them. *The problem cannot be the game,* we tell ourselves. *The problem must be with those bad men who have been indulged all their lives because of their athletic talents. They are bad. The game is good.* Our conformational intelligence and cognitive dissonance will not let us accept any other explanation.

It is time we admit the truth. The New Testament book of Romans tells us, "Do not conform yourself to this age but be transformed by the renewal of your mind, that you may discern what is the will of God, what is good and pleasing and perfect."[1] This is what we must do. We must allow truth to transform our minds and change the way we see the world around us. I wrote this book to bring the truth to light. Now that you know the truth, you must act upon it. It is not enough to just be aware of the truth. In America, we do many things to raise awareness. Driving down the street, I see pink ribbon magnets on the backs of cars to raise awareness for breast cancer, and yellow ribbons to raise awareness for our troops overseas. January is National Codependency Awareness month, while April is Autism Awareness month and Sexual Assault Awareness month, and the list goes on and on and on. We set aside months and have symbols to raise awareness for anything and everything.

But awareness is not the same as action.

The country of my birth was embroiled in a bitter civil war when I came into this world. Stories about the crisis in Biafra made worldwide headlines. News magazines like *Life* and *Time* featured photographs of starving children in Biafra. Yes, the world was aware of the plight of my nation and my people. I was one of those children, born malnourished. Only by the grace of God did I survive until the end of the war. The world knew all about the crisis through which I lived. But the world did nothing. Awareness is not enough, for, as God's Word teaches us, "wisdom is vindicated by her works."[2]

When you become aware of the truth, you must act upon it. Only by taking action can the truth truly set us free. So what action do you need to take in response to all you have read in these pages?

First, value your brain. Your mind and your memories make you who you are. Treasure your mind. Protect your brain. Do not take your mental health for granted. Take steps to protect it.

Second, protect the brains of your children. Do not allow your underage children (younger than eighteen years old) to engage in high-impact, high-contact sports, which can cause brain trauma and brain damage. Take precautions in other less-impact, less-contact sports, as well as in noncontact sports where incidental and accidental brain trauma may occur. I tell soccer parents everywhere, "Do not let your children do headers, and do not let them play soccer or lacrosse until they are about twelve to fourteen years old." If you are involved in a soccer league as a parent or coach, help pass rules that will take headers out of the game for children under eighteen. The best and most appropriate sports for children under the age of eighteen are the noncollision, nonimpact, noncontact sports.

Third, let us love one another, for love is of God.[3] To love my fellow human being means I see them for who they truly are—a person made in the image of the living God. Too often our sports heroes are not human beings in our eyes. They are gladiators, putting their bodies and minds at risk for our entertainment. When I begin to see them through the eyes of God, I cannot continue to be a party to their pain. I simply cannot.

•　•　•　•

May we always have the grace and wisdom to know when we are called to stand by the truth, to fight battles in defense of the truth and light, no matter how insignificant and inconsequential we may think our lives are. God is the only truth and light, and the truth does not take sides. And in Him and by Him, all things are possible in our lives; the impossible becomes possible, if we only believe. And let us act on our beliefs and act on the truth. Let us do the little, good things in life—one person at a time, one act at a time—to improve the lot of all our fellow human beings. Together, our small acts add up to become a force that improves the lot of all of us and all mankind. We are all members of one another; what happens to the least of us, happens to all of us.

Bennet Omalu
Lodi, California

Questions from Parents about Brain Trauma and Contact Sports, Especially Football

What are some recent discoveries affecting junior football play?

A child can suffer permanent brain damage from playing football, even after only one season of football, without suffering any concussion. The cause of brain damage is less about concussions but more about repeated blows to the head —with or without concussions, with or without helmets. The younger you are when you begin to play, the greater the risk of permanent brain damage and the greater the risk of cumulative exposure to brain damage. Even a single documented concussion can cause brain damage. Studies have shown that if a child plays a high-impact, high-contact sport like football, that child stands a higher risk of dropping out of high school, not attending college, not doing well in life, becoming reliant upon the social welfare system and dependent on disability payouts as an adult, developing psychiatric and psychological problems later in life, receiving drug prescriptions for psychiatric illnesses, and even dying at a younger age.

Just how much damage can happen and when? Even at an early age?

Significant damage can happen any time and at any age. We do not know the exact blow—or how many blows—that will cause permanent brain damage. Anyone who plays football has a 100 percent risk exposure to permanent brain damage. There is no such thing as a safe blow or impact to the human head, just like there is no such thing as safe cigarette smoking. Every blow and impact to the human head can be dangerous. God did not intend for us to play games like football when He created our heads and brains. The younger a child is when he or she plays football or other high-impact, high-contact sports, the greater the risk of cumulative brain damage.

What sports do make a lot of sense to play?

Adults are free to play any sport they want to play, no matter how dangerous. It is within the rights, free will, freedom, and liberty of every adult to choose to play any sport and engage in any activity he or she wants to play or engage in. This is not about adults, but about our children.

Children should engage in sports that are noncontact or less contact. For an enumeration of available noncontact sports that are brain-friendlier, visit the website of the International Olympics Committee (IOC) at www .olympic.org. I did that when it was time for my children, Ashly and Mark, to play sports. Today they play brain-friendly games that are noncontact, including track and field sports, badminton, volleyball, table tennis, baseball, basketball, swimming, and kick-only, less-dribble soccer. No contact sports for them. True sports are meant to be recreational and rejuvenating. True sports are meant to build up the child who plays them and not destroy that child and rob that child of what defines him or her as a human being—his or her mind and intellect. Having watched the Olympics every four years, I know that brain-friendly noncontact sports can be as entertaining and as exciting as contact sports. Moving forward into the twenty-first century, our children should engage in sports that build up their brains rather than destroy them.

Less-impact, less-contact sports like soccer may be permissible. In these types of sports, incidental blows to the head do occur, but they are not intrinsic to the play of the game. I believe modifications should be made to these games as we play them today to make them safer for our children. Specifically, in soccer for children, we should eliminate heading of the ball; make the ball softer, lighter, and slightly bigger; and reduce the number of players on each team in order to reduce the number of players on the field at the same time—therefore reducing the risk of players running into each other by accident. Playing less-impact, less-contact sports like soccer requires adequate development of brain functioning for reflexes and coordination, which the brains of children have not attained developmentally. Therefore, we can increase the age limit for children to participate in these games. For example, children may not be allowed to play dribble soccer until they are twelve or fourteen years old to give them a chance to attain adequate development of brain reflexes and coordination. Before then, they may engage in less-dribble, less-contact kick-soccer.

If I choose to put my kids in football, is there any advice you can offer based on what you've learned about sports?

I really do not have any advice about what to do if your child is playing football. The only advice I have for a parent about football is that if your child is younger than eighteen years old, please do not let him or her play football or other high-impact, high-contact sports. It is not worth the risk. If your child plays football, he has a 100 percent risk exposure to brain injury and brain damage. There is no helmet on the market that will eliminate this risk. Your child can wait until he or she turns eighteen years old—just like your child can wait until he or she turns eighteen or twenty-one years old to smoke or drink or join the military. I do not let my children play, so if I were to advise other parents to allow their children to play, it would be unethical for me, and I would be falling short of my duties as a Christian and my call to love and treat my neighbor as I would treat myself. If your child is already playing football or other high-impact, high-contact sports, please stop them today. Stopping their brain from receiving the next blow may be the very thing that will save them.

What about the whole effort to limit play to *game* tackling only, not in practice?

It does not make any difference. Limiting tackling only to games still exposes your child to repeated blows to the head. The fundamental issue is not about concussions but about repeated blows to the head, no matter how seemingly innocuous those blows could be. Your child can still suffer brain damage, even after only one season of playing football, without suffering any concussions. In the management of risk, if you identify a risk, you mitigate exposure to that risk and eliminate that risk, if and when possible. Football is not an indispensable activity of daily living like transportation; we do not need sports like football to live, and therefore they should be avoided and eliminated for our children. There are so many other alternative sports for them to engage in. An analogy is cigarette smoking. We have identified cigarette smoking to be dangerous, just like we have identified blows to the head in any activity to be dangerous. We do not advise any child to smoke only one cigarette a day (or five cigarettes a day) as opposed to an entire pack. All cigarette smoking is dangerous, just like every blow to the head is dangerous. Repeated blows to the head over time can even be more dangerous for a child than smoking half a cigarette a day—yet we do not allow children to smoke, but we allow them to suffer traumatic brain injury. In most jurisdictions in the United States, the intentional and sometimes unintentional exposure of a child to the risk of serious bodily harm and pain qualifies as child abuse or neglect. The injury does not have to occur for you to be in violation of the law. For example, if you leave your seven-year-old child alone at home and you go to work, you can lose custody of that child solely because you left that child home alone. But in allowing your child to play football, you are even doing something worse for them. We are choosing to intentionally expose our children to the risk of permanent brain damage from high-impact, high-contact sports like football. This is simply not the right thing to do, especially if you love your children, like all of us parents do.

Do studies show that concussion helmets, if worn throughout a player's career, will help prevent concussions?

No. Helmets do not prevent subconcussions and concussions. Helmets prevent abrasions, contusions, and lacerations of your face and scalp; fractures of your skull; and bleeding inside your skull. They do not prevent your brain from bouncing around inside your skull and impacting the inner surfaces. Helmets may actually increase the risk of your child suffering subconcussions and concussions. Your child is more likely to hit with his helmet because he feels less or no pain. There is no skin-to-skin contact. The helmet also increases the weight and size of your child's head and increases the momentum of the impacts and the amounts of energy that reach your child's brain and cause brain injury. Helmets are not the answer. The only answer at this time is prevention. The brain floats freely inside the skull, and nothing on the outside of the skull and scalp will stop the brain from moving and bouncing around the skull.

What about flag or touch football?

I do not know much about touch or flag football. If either involves the same blows to the head as regular football, they are not safe. As I understand them, touch and flag football are designed to be noncontact games, which make them a safe alternative to full-contact football. However, I do know that in touch and flag football, opposing teams line up against each other, and when they play, the players still do have collisions as part of the play. I caution parents against allowing their children to play football in any form. Noncontact forms of the game feed the illusion that football in all forms is safe while also building a stronger desire for a child to play full-contact football in middle school or high school. I have already addressed the dangers that this poses.

At what age does CTE set in?

CTE can set in at any age. Symptoms can begin at any age. Subtle symptoms may first manifest themselves while your child is playing and may go unnoticed. Sometimes it can take up to forty years for your child to exhibit serious and incapacitating symptoms. This can happen after your child has stopped playing and has long forgotten that he played. CTE is not the only danger. There is also another disease called PTE (Post-Traumatic Encephalopathy) that can also manifest during or after your child has stopped playing. One of the commonest types of PTE is Post-Traumatic Epilepsy. The long-term effects of blows to the head encompass a spectrum and continuum of diseases that involve physical brain damage, inflammation of the brain, and impaired functioning of the brain that may not always end up in either CTE or PTE, which are the more advanced and more permanent forms of this spectrum of diseases.

Have you done studies on the college and high school level, and have you seen CTE take effect in younger athletes?

Yes, I have seen CTE and PTE in teenagers and athletes in their early twenties. I have also seen ALS (amyotrophic lateral sclerosis—Lou Gehrig's disease) in children who played football and developed the disease in their twenties and thirties. When they develop ALS, it is a form of CTE involving the spinal cord (CTE-ALS). The predominant symptoms are motor symptoms and movement disorders.

Does the brain injury have to be repetitive to cause CTE?

No, brain injuries do not have to be repetitive to cause CTE. CTE can occur outside of sports as a result of domestic violence, physical abuse of children, motor vehicle accidents, domestic accidents, other industrial and occupational accidents, physical assaults, and exposure to explosives, like in military veterans. But in sports, you are more likely to have the scenario of repetitive impacts to the head, which cause subconcussive and concussive injuries that can become cumulative over time. In subconcussive injuries, you will have injuries on the microscopic cellular level without any obvious and incapacitating symptoms. Concussive injuries display obvious and sometimes incapacitating symptoms, which can be transient. Subconcussive and concussive injuries are more prevalent in high-impact, high-contact sports, are cumulative in nature, and over time result in cumulative and permanent injuries. Therefore, every blow to the head is of a forensically consequential nature. This is why parents who have the habit of smacking or knocking their children on the head as admonishment should stop that—as well as *all* forms of domestic violence. Every blow to the head can be dangerous.

How do you think the NFL changes will affect CTE? Have they gone far enough?

No, the NFL has not gone far enough. The changes that have been made still do not remove the head from the game. In fact, I do not think that football as we play it today can ever be made safe, just like boxing cannot be made safe. The NFL has instituted new guidelines for concussion management, but the fundamental issue is not about concussions but about repeated blows to the head. The NFL guidelines should be about each and every blow to the head while playing football, but the league will not recognize that, because in so doing, they will have to admit that football is inherently dangerous. Even with the new concussion protocols and guidelines, once a player has suffered a concussion, the damage to the brain has occurred. The new guidelines cannot reverse that damage. There is no cure for a concussion, although the symptoms of a concussion may be treated. But the damage done to the brain by a concussion cannot be reversed or cured, especially within the context of repeated blows to the head. What do we have to do? We must recognize the truth for what it is, for there can only be one truth—and based on the truth, we become empowered and enlightened to discover solutions and cures. A solution cannot be derived if we do not recognize and accept the one truth.

What is the safest position a child can play in football?

There is no "safest" position a child can play in football. Debilitating brain injuries have been found in every position on the football field—from linemen and offensive and defensive backs to kickers and punters. Every position on the field puts a child at risk. Stating that there is a safe position a child can play in football is like stating that there are a certain number of cigarettes a day a child can safely smoke. Potentially dangerous activities should be left for adults who have reached the age of consent. Every position in football is dangerous for a child. A child is anyone under the age of eighteen, and this is when your child's brain begins to become fully developed as an adult. The human brain becomes fully developed from about eighteen to twenty-five years old.

Have you found any differences in positions played and the connection to CTE?

Research data has shown that players who play certain positions are more likely to receive a greater number of blows to their heads. However, there are many more factors involved that have nothing to do with the position you play—for example, the style of play of the player. A more aggressive player, regardless of the position played, is more likely to be injured than a less aggressive player. Every player who plays every position in football has a 100 percent risk exposure to repeated blows to the head and to brain trauma—with or without a helmet, with or without concussions—and can develop permanent brain damage, CTE, and PTE over time.

I thought that children could regenerate brain tissue. Can't that help children be safe from CTE?

The human brain does not have any reasonable capacity to regenerate itself. We are born with a finite number of brain cells. We can only lose our brain cells; we cannot create new ones. There has been an experimental proposition of limited stem cells in the brain—and that some of these stem cells may be instigated and programmed to create new brain cells—but these propositions remain at academic and experimental laboratory levels that have no reasonable applications in actual patients and in real life. As physicians and healers, we need to be empathetic, truthful, hopeful, and sincere with patients and not give false hopes to children and their families. We have more brain cells than we may actually need, so we have high compensatory and rehabilitative capacities for neurological functioning, especially in children, who are more likely to have greater temporal re-serves. However, the brains of children are still developing and establishing the neural interconnectivity and architecture that developed adult brains have. Brain trauma affects this developing neural interconnectivity and architecture in children and makes their brains more vulnerable to brain trauma than the brains of adults.

Is there a way to reverse CTE?

As of today, given where we are in medical science and science in general, permanent brain damage from all types of brain trauma cannot be reversed. CTE and PTE cannot be reversed. The only cure is prevention. During and after brain trauma, medical care can control the degree and extent of damage, but it cannot reverse it or cure it.

In what other sports have you found CTE?

There is a risk of developing CTE in every high-impact, high-contact sport where repeated blows to the head are prevalent, where blows to the head are intrinsic to the play of the game. The most notorious high-impact, high-contact sports are football, ice hockey, boxing, wrestling, mixed martial arts, and rugby. CTE has also been found in BMX bikers, as well as in soccer players as a result of headers and accidental collision injuries. That is why, in my opinion, headers should be removed from youth soccer, and children younger than twelve to fourteen years old should not play dribble-soccer or lacrosse as we play them today. Given the physiological differences between boys and girls, men and women, some of these contact sports may have to be modified for girls in order to lower the high risk of exposure to concussions like we have in women's soccer.

Is there any way to diagnose CTE while an athlete/person is living?

A presumptive diagnosis of CTE can be made by a physician based on the constellation of symptoms and signs, medical history, and history of exposure to brain trauma. The key word is "presumptive" diagnosis, which means a reasonable degree (greater than 50 percent) of certainty. However, *definitive* diagnosis, with 100 percent certainty, can only be done after the patient dies and the brain tissue is examined. These standards also apply to dementias such as Alzheimer's disease. So the answer is yes, if you believe you have symptoms of CTE, you should go see a physician who specializes in the diagnosis and treatment of all types of brain damage caused by brain trauma. These types of physicians include neurologists, psychiatrists, and physicians who specialize in physical medicine and rehabilitation. I must reiterate that neuropsychiatric testing—evaluating a brain trauma patient with psychological testing—should not be used to diagnose CTE or brain trauma. The FDA does not approve the use of neuropsychiatric tests for the diagnosis of brain trauma or CTE. Neuropsychiatric testing is used to monitor cognitive functioning, and it should stop at that. Parents have been systematically misled to believe that neuropsychiatric testing (imPACT testing, for example) is the answer to brain trauma in sports. This is not true. Once a child has suffered a concussion or another type of brain trauma in sports, there is actually nothing a neuropsychiatric test does for that child.

Are brain scans/MRIs effective in diagnosing CTE?

There is currently no brain scan that has been approved by the Food and Drug Administration for the definitive diagnosis of CTE. Experimentally, using various modalities of brain scans, there are changes that we are observing in brains of patients with permanent brain damage, CTE, and PTE.

What is the treatment for CTE (assuming that a determination/ diagnosis can be made pre-death)?

The treatment of CTE when it is presumptively diagnosed in a living person involves symptomatic relief and long-term management. As of today, there is no cure for CTE.

Are you suggesting that the only way to prevent CTE is less-contact or noncontact sports?

Yes. As a physician and epidemiologist who has been involved in the investigation of more than twelve thousand deaths, I am convinced that there is a God, and as human beings, *we* cannot be God. We cannot create life, and we can never have all the answers for all the questions that exist in our lives. As of today, medicine as a science does not have the cure for many diseases, not even a cure for diseases as common as strokes. The brain does not have any reasonable ability or capacity to regenerate itself. A brain cell does not divide to create a new brain cell and regenerate the brain. This is where we are today. Death of brain tissue from all types of injuries is permanent. Based on where we are as human beings in our faith journey and in our science, the only way to prevent CTE is to avoid blows to the head in every human activity. This is why volitional exposure of a child to the risk of any type of brain injury is not the wise thing to do in the twenty-first century for our children.

Is shaken baby syndrome basically CTE? Does it present the same issues?

In the world of forensic pathology, shaken baby syndrome is now known as non-accidental trauma (NAT) in a child. In non-accidental trauma, the child can suffer severe abusive head injuries. All types of severe head injuries can cause permanent and irreversible brain damage, which can manifest as CTE or PTE later in life.

What are the symptoms of CTE?

CTE can manifest with a broad variety of symptoms, which can be divided into cognitive, behavioral, and mood disorders. Symptoms may begin immediately and persist permanently. Symptoms may abate significantly, but residual symptoms may persist permanently. Symptoms may improve over time. Symptoms may not manifest over a long, delayed period, sometimes up to forty years, but begin to manifest in a subtle but progressive manner. Symptoms may go unnoticed, but when a physician tests the child or adult, symptoms will be elicited. The cognitive symptoms may include, but are not limited to, loss of memory or memory impairment; diminishing intelligence or loss of intelligence; impaired ability to study and learn or to assimilate new knowledge and information; inability to engage in complex, derivative, or extrapolative reasoning and thinking; inability to engage in executive functioning; and impaired language capacity and functioning. The behavioral symptoms may include, but are not limited to, impaired ability to focus on tasks and remain attentive for long periods; increasing tendency to engage in criminal and violent behavior; increasing impulsivity; increasing irrational risk-taking behavior, paranoid behavior, sexual improprieties, and aggression; disinhibition and loss of learned behavior and social decencies; chronic alcoholism; chronic drug abuse; inability to obtain, sustain, and maintain jobs; impaired financial functioning and bankruptcies; and impaired ability to maintain and sustain intimate relationships. The mood disorders may include, but are not limited to, major depression; rampant fluctuations in mood from highs to lows, and lows to highs; exaggerated reactions to daily life stressors; impaired ability to control emotions and drives; and suicidal behavior, suicidal ideations, suicidal attempts, and completed suicides. Other physical symptoms may include insomnia; inability to fall asleep and stay asleep; headaches and migraines; impairment of motor functioning; and movement disorders that may resemble amyotrophic lateral sclerosis (ALS) or Parkinson's disease. Not every patient will manifest with all these symptoms, and not every patient will manifest the same way. Symptoms may range from negligible, mild, moderate, severe, and marked to debilitating.

Are seizures a sign of brain damage?

All types of brain injury can cause permanent physical damage to the brain, which can manifest as PTE or CTE. One of the most prevalent types of PTE is Post-Traumatic Epilepsy. Therefore, seizures can follow all types of brain injury. I have personally encountered several football players who suffer from Post-Traumatic Epilepsy.

If I have played football but stopped and have never suffered a concussion, am I still at risk for contracting CTE?

Yes, you are still at risk of suffering CTE later in life. The cause of CTE is not concussions but blows to the head. Each and every blow to your head you receive while playing football—with or without a helmet, with or without a concussion—increases your risk of suffering permanent brain damage, which can manifest as CTE later in your life. Concussions do not cause brain damage; blows to the head do. Concussion is a disease by itself, which is an outcome or product of a blow to the head and belongs to the spectrum of diseases caused by blows to the head, which we now call the Traumatic Encephalopathy Syndromes. The spectrum of diseases following brain trauma and brain damage is not limited to just CTE and PTE. CTE and PTE also belong to the Traumatic Encephalopathy Syndromes.

Are the injuries/CTE from getting hit or doing the hitting the same?

The two are the same. No matter whether you are getting hit or doing the hitting, your helmeted head is sustaining blunt force trauma, and your brain is sustaining repeated subconcussive and concussive injuries. However, the person who is hit and is not aware he or she is being hit may be more likely to suffer angular-rotational-acceleration-deceleration injuries of the brain, which may be more dangerous

Are you happy with the changes you are seeing in the NFL and in other sports?

No, I am not satisfied with the changes I am seeing in the NFL and in other sports. It remains disheartening to me that executives and physicians of these sports organizations still deny that football, ice hockey, wrestling, mixed martial arts, and other high-impact, high-contact sports can cause permanent brain damage. The changes that have been made do not address the fundamental issue of exposure of the human head and brain to repeated blows. The focus has been on concussions, which is a misappropriation of the science. Concussions do not cause brain damage; blows to the head do. Concussion is a disease by itself, which is an outcome or product of a blow to the head and belongs to the spectrum of diseases caused by blows to the head. Once a concussion has occurred, the injury is permanent; it cannot be cured. The symptoms may abate, but the brain remembers the concussion in a cumulative manner over time. Therefore, there are no changes made by the NFL or other leagues that will adequately address the risk of brain injury in football, ice hockey, boxing, wrestling, mixed martial arts, rugby, and other high-impact, high-contact sports like BMX biking. Boxing can never be made safe. Football as we play it today can never be made safe. Skydiving can never be made safe. This is why my position has always been that for adults, we can play these games as much as we want without any reservation whatsoever. I will be one of the first to stand up to defend the right of an adult to exercise his or her individual rights, free will, freedom, and liberty to play any game he or she wants to play—*but not for our children*. It is our moral duty as a society to protect our children from all types of harm and to help every child reach his or her God-given intellectual and cognitive capacities. Brain injuries suffered while playing football, ice hockey, and other high-impact, high-contact sports steal away the gift of life from our children. Given my position, only children eighteen years old and older should play football as we play it today. This means we can still enjoy college football and NFL football as we play and enjoy them today!

What is the one thing you would like parents to know about their children and CTE?

Every parent who loves and cherishes their children and recognizes that the gift of life is the greatest gift of all must not allow any child to play high-impact, high-contact sports like boxing, football, ice hockey, mixed martial arts, wrestling, and rugby. Caution should be exercised when your child plays the less-contact, less-impact sports such as soccer and lacrosse, which must be modified for our children as well. When you allow your child to engage in these contact sports, you are exposing him or her to the risk of permanent brain damage, which can manifest as CTE. CTE steals away that gift of life from your child and can permanently ruin your child's life when he or she becomes a teenager or a young adult. Our children should play only less-impact and less-contact sports or noncontact sports until they turn eighteen and become adults, at which point they can do whatever they want to do, including joining the military and playing high-impact, high-contact sports. The fundamental issue is not concussions but repeated blows to the head—with or without concussions, with or without helmets. We must mitigate the exposure of our children's brains to all types of blows to the head in all types of sports and in all types of human activities. We must be cautious when our children play the less-impact and less-contact sports. I believe noncontact sports are safest for our children.

What age is appropriate for playing tackle football?

There is no age that is appropriate for playing tackle football, just like there is no age that is appropriate for smoking. However, adults have the right, free will, freedom, and liberty to do whatever they want to do—as long as it does not cause injury to or undermine the safety of another person. But when it comes to children, we need to protect them from all things that have the potential to cause harm to them, and tackle football is one of them, just like smoking and child abuse and neglect are.

Is hockey safer than football for high schoolers?

Ice hockey is a high-impact, high-contact sports and is as dangerous as football. Other dangerous high-impact, high-contact sports that can damage the brain are football, rugby, boxing, wrestling, and mixed martial arts.

Acknowledgments

To my collaborator, Mark Tabb, and my literary agent, Steve Ross—thank you so much for believing in me, inspiring me to step forward, and supporting me to write this book. I am deeply grateful. I give you credit for this book, for without you two, there would not have been this book. May God continue to bless you most abundantly.

To all the angels in my life, through whom I received God's blessings:

- my father, John Omalu; my mother, Caroline Omalu; my brothers and sisters, Onyi, Winny, Uche, Ikem, Chizoba, and Mie-Mie. You are my essence.
- my in-laws, Sam, Chuma, Ibe, Chineme, Loretta, Nneka, Mummy, Susan, John, and Tom. You have enriched our lives immeasurably
- my uncle, Remy
- my teachers, who were the wind beneath my wings—Dr. Carlos Navarro, Dr. Cyril Wecht, Dr. Ronald Hamilton, Dr. Abdulrezak Shakir, and Dr. Clayton Wiley
- Jeanne Marie Laskas, who was the angel to first tell the world about me and who did me justice
- my agents, Don Epstein, Elyse Cheney, and Matthew Snyder, who guided me and kept me out of trouble
- Andy Ward, you are a true leader
- my Hollywood family—Peter Landesman, Will Smith, Jada Smith, Gugu Mbatha-Raw, David Wolthoff, Larry Shuman, Ridley Scott, Giannina Scott, Amal Bagger, Albert Brooks, David Morse, Mike

O'Malley, Hill Harper, Adewale Akinnuoye-Agbaje, and every cast and crew member of the movie *Concussion*. You have made me who I am, and I remain deeply grateful and indebted to you. May God bless you most abundantly and grant you your hearts' desires.

Peter and Will, you did such a phenomenal job. You said you would do me justice—and yes, you really did! Words cannot express what gratitude I have inside me for what you have done for me. You lifted me up when I was down and out in the cold, and you invited me in to the warmth of your hearts. I now take you two as my brothers. My family is deeply grateful to you for honoring my father and placing his picture in the movie.

David Wolthoff, I am simply dumbfounded when it comes to you. You believed in my story when no one else would. You kept the faith in me and continued pushing on. Simply put, there would have been no movie without you. I am profoundly grateful, David. Together we shall continue doing great things.

To my Sony Pictures family—Tom Rothman, Amy Pascal, Doug Belgrad, Elizabeth Cantillon, Jennifer Mcgrath, Elena Russell-Nava, and every Sony employee who worked on *Concussion*, especially during the promotion. I had fun, and you took very good care of me. Without you, my story would not have been told. You extended a hand of friendship to me, pulled me up, and helped mold me into what I am today. I remain deeply grateful to you.

To Father Carmen D'Amico and my St. Benedict the Moor parish family in Pittsburgh, you guided me to the light of Christ and empowered my faith. I am deeply grateful. Without you, I may not have discovered the preeminence of God in all things visible and invisible.

To my Greater Talent Network family—David, Jennifer, Kristine, Jillian, and every staff member I have worked with—you lifted me up and made me shine. I am deeply grateful. To my San Joaquin County family, the board of supervisors; every county coworker who serves our county, especially at the district attorney's office, the sheriff's office, and the San

Joaquin General Hospital, I count myself deeply lucky and honored to serve with you. I am deeply thankful for all your support. Together may we continue to bring good light upon our county. Tori, Steve, Deepak, Sue, Annette, Barbara, Lek, Micky, Toby, Mike, Dan, Jose, Frankie, Ted, Etta, Kathryn, and Alex—on a daily basis, you are the struts that keep me standing. I am deeply thankful.

To my University of California, Davis family, Dr. Lydia Howell and Dr. Ralph Green—you gave me an academic home and supported me when everyone else looked away. I am deeply grateful.

To my friends, Bob Fitzsimmons, Jimmy Adegoke, Obinna Okoye, Jennifer Hammers, and Julian Bailes, thank you so much for the support you have given me. Your friendship has been a source of tremendous grace and peace to me. May God bless you most abundantly.

To Mike Webster, Terry Long, Andre Waters, Justin Strzelczyk, Chris Benoit, Fred McNeill, and every other athlete and military veteran I met in death in the search of the truth and light of our faith and science, I honor you and thank you for teaching us so much with your lives. Together we shall prevent yet another child, man, or woman from suffering what you suffered. Thank you so much for the enlightenment you offered us in your death and for glorifying the truth.

To everyone else—especially every person I should have mentioned but could not mention because of the limitation of space in this book—whose paths have crossed with mine, I want you to know that all I feel in my heart is love, the love of us all as one family of mankind. May we all continue to enjoy that peace of our oneness. I wish you every happiness and joy.

Notes

Chapter 2: Child of War

1. Mathew 5:14–16.

Chapter 5: "Heaven Is Here, and America Is Here"

1. Isaiah 43:18–21.

Chapter 7: Through the Wilderness

1. Hebrews 11:1.

Chapter 11: A Divine Appointment

1. As of this writing I've performed more than eight thousand autopsies and participated in the investigation of more than ten thousand death cases.

Chapter 13: A Game-Changing Diagnosis

1. Cited in Mark Fainaru-Wada and Steve Fainaru, *League of Denial: The NFL, Concussions, and the Battle for Truth* (New York: Random House, 2014), 138.
2. Ibid., 57.

Chapter 14: Nearly Over before It Begins

1. Mathew 18:20.
2. John 11:22.
3. John 14:13–14.
4. John 15:7.
5. John 15:16.
6. John 16:23.

Chapter 15: The NFL = Big Tobacco

1. From the 1993 case *Daubert v. Merrell Dow Pharmaceuticals*.
2. See Mark J. Denger and Norman S. Marshall, "Californians and the Military:

Admiral Joseph Mason 'Bull' Reeves, USN," www.militarymuseum.org/Reeves.html (accessed February 1, 2017).

3. "Competitive athletics: a statement of policy: report of the Committee on School Health, American Academy of Pediatrics," *Pennsylvania Medical Journal* 60.5 (May 1957): 627–29.

4. Laura Purcell, MD, and Claire M. A. LaBlanc, MD, "Policy Statement—Boxing Participation by Children and Adolescents," American Academy of Pediatrics, Council on Sports Medicine and Fitness, Canadian Paediatric Society, Healthy Active Living and Sports Medicine Committee, *Pediatrics* 128.3 (September 2011): 617–23.

5. Elliot J. Pellman et al., "Concussion in Professional Football: Repeat Injuries—Part 4," *Neurosurgery* 55.4 (October 2004): 870, www.researchgate.net/publication/8256145_Concussion_in_Professional_Football_Repeat_Injuries -Part_4 (accessed February 1, 2017).

6. Ibid.

7. Ibid.

8. See Elliot Pellman et al., "Concussion in Professional Football: Players Returning to the Same Game—Part 7," *Neurosurgery* 56.1 (January 2005): 79–92, www .researchgate.net/publication/8112277_Concussion_in_professional_football _Players_returning_to_the_same_game_-_Part_7 (accessed February 1, 2017).

9. Anders Hambérger et al., "Concussion in Professional Football: Morphology of Brain Injuries in the NFL Concussion Model—Part 16," *Neurosurgery* 64.6 (June 2009): 1174, https://www.researchgate.net/publication/26258655_Concussion _in_professional_football_Morphology_of_brain_injuries_in_the_NFL _concussion_model_-_Part_16 (accessed February 1, 2017).

10. Mark Maske, "Cowboys Owner Jerry Jones: 'Absurd' to Think Current Data Shows Clear Link between CTE, Football," *Washington Post*, March 23, 2016, www.washingtonpost.com/news/sports/wp/2016/03/22/jerry-jones-does -not-believe-a-link-between-football-and-brain-disease-has-been-established (accessed February 1, 2017).

11. Zak Keefer, "Colts Owner Jim Irsay on Concussions: 'No One Knew Anything,'" *Indianapolis Star*, March 28, 2016, www.indystar.com/story/sports/nfl/colts/2016/03/28/colts-owner-jim-irsay-concussions-no-one-knew -anything/82341376 (accessed February 1, 2017).

Chapter 16: "In the Name of Christ, Stop!"

1. The story is told by Theodoret of Cyrus in *The Ecclesiastical History*, Book V, Chapter XXVI ("Of Honorius the emperor and Telemachus the monk"), www .newadvent.org/fathers/27025.htm (accessed February 1, 2017).

2. Bennet I. Omalu et al., "Fatal Fulminant Pan-Meningo-Polioencephalitis Due to West Nile Virus," *Brain Pathology* 13.4 (October 2003): 465–72, www.mailman

.columbia.edu/sites/default/files/legacy/fatalfulminantpan-meningo-polio encephalitisduetowestnilevirus.pdf (accessed February 17, 2017).

3. H. B. Armah, G. Wang, B. I. Omalu et al., "Systemic Distribution of West Nile Virus Infection: Postmortem Immunohistochemical Study of Six Cases," *Brain Pathology* 17.4 (October 2007): 354–62.

4. B. I. Omalu et al., "Chronic Traumatic Encephalopathy in a National Football League Player," *Neurosurgery* 57.1 (July 2005): 132, www.jeannemarielaskas.com/ wp-content/uploads/2015/10/CTE-NFL-part-1.pdf (accessed February 1, 2017).

5. Romans 8:28, 31, 35, 37–39.

Chapter 17: The Baton Is Passed

1. Ira R. Casson, Elliot J. Pellman, and David C. Viano, "Chronic Traumatic Encephalopathy in a National Football League Player: To the Editor," *Neurosurgery* 58.5 (May 2006): E1003, http://journals.lww.com/neurosurgery/ Fulltext/2006/05000/Chronic_Traumatic_Encephalopathy_in_a_National.35 .aspx (accessed February 1, 2017).

2. Ed Bouchette, "Surgeon Disagrees with Wecht That Football Killed Long," *Pittsburgh Post-Gazette*, September 15, 2005, www.post-gazette.com/sports/ steelers/2005/09/15/Surgeon-disagrees-with-Wecht-that-football-killed-Long/ stories/200509150517 (accessed February 1, 2017).

3. Bennet I. Omalu et al., "Chronic Traumatic Encephalopathy in a National Football League Player: To the Editor: In Reply," *Neurosurgery* 58.5 (May 2006): E1003, http://journals.lww.com/neurosurgery/Fulltext/2006/05000/Chronic _Traumatic_Encephalopathy_in_a_National.36.aspx (accessed February 1, 2017).

4. Donald W. Marion, "Chronic Traumatic Encephalopathy in a National Football League Player: To the Editor: In Reply," *Neurosurgery* 58.5 (May 2006): E1003, http://journals.lww.com/neurosurgery/Fulltext/2006/05000/Chronic _Traumatic_Encephalopathy_in_a_National.41.aspx (accessed February 1, 2017).

5. Robert Dvorchak, "Wecht: Long Died from Brain Injury: Had Head Trauma from NFL Days," *Pittsburgh Post-Gazette*, September 14, 2005, www.post -gazette.com/sports/steelers/2005/09/14/Wecht-Long-died-from-brain-injury/ stories/200509140347 (accessed February 1, 2017).

6. Quoted in Ed Bouchette, "Surgeon Disagrees with Wecht That Football Killed Long," *Pittsburgh Post-Gazette*, September 15, 2005, www.post-gazette .com/sports/steelers/2005/09/15/Surgeon-disagrees-with-Wecht-that-football -killed-Long/stories/200509150517 (accessed February 1, 2017); Jonathan Silver, "Suicide Ruling in Long's Death Hasn't Ended Controversy," *Pittsburgh Post-Gazette*, January 26, 2006, http://www.post-gazette.com/sports/ steelers/2006/01/26/Suicide-ruling-in-Long-s-death-hasn-t-ended-controversy/ stories/200601260352 (accessed February 1, 2017).

7. Paula Reed Ward, "Wecht Indicted by Grand Jury: Medical Examiner Accused of Public Use, Private Gain," *Pittsburgh Post-Gazette*, January 21, 2006, 1,

8. Paula Reed Ward, "Wecht Charges Dropped: Forensic Pathologist Call Buchanan 'a Sore Loser,'" June 3, 2009, *Pittsburgh Post-Gazette*, www.post-gazette.com/local/region/2009/06/03/Wecht-charges-dropped/stories/200906030214 (accessed February 1, 2017).

9. Steve Almasy and Jill Martin, "Judge Approves NFL Concussion Lawsuit Settlement," *CNN*, April 22, 2015, www.cnn.com/2015/04/22/us/nfl-concussion-lawsuit-settlement (accessed February 1, 2017); Christian Red, "Supreme Court Ruling Paves Way for NFL Retirees to Receive Concussion Benefits," *New York Daily News*, December 12, 2016, www.nydailynews.com/sports/football/nfl-1-billion-concussion-settlement-approved-supreme-court-article-1.2908003 (accessed February 1, 2017).

10. See Robert Dvorchak, "Steelers Doctor Says Concluding Football Led to Long's Demise Is Bad Science," *Pittsburgh Post-Gazette*, September 16, 2005, www.post-gazette.com/sports/steelers/2005/09/16/Steelers-doctor-says-concluding-football-led-to-Long-s-demise-is-bad-science/stories/200509160237 (accessed February 1, 2017).

11. "FDA Allows Marketing of First-of-Kind Computerized Cognitive Tests to Help Assess Cognitive Skills after a Head Injury," FDA News Release, August 22, 2016, www.fda.gov/NewsEvents/Newsroom/PressAnnouncements/ucm517526.htm (accessed February 1, 2017).

12. Bennet I. Omalu et al., "Chronic Traumatic Encephalopathy in a National Football League Player: Part II," *Neurosurgery* 59.5 (November 2006): 1086–93, https://www.researchgate.net/publication/6656243_Chronic_traumatic_encephalopathy_in_a_National_Football_League_player_Part_II (accessed February 1, 2017).

13. David C. Viano, "Concussion in Professional Football: Performance of Newer Helmets in Reconstructed Game Impacts," *Neurosurgery* 59.3 (September 2006): 591–606, https://www.researchgate.net/publication/6962379_Concussion_in_Professional_Football_Performance_of_Newer_Helmets_in_Reconstructed_Game_ImpactsPart_13 (accessed February 1, 2017).

14. Alan Schwarz, "Expert Ties Ex-Player's Suicide to Brain Damage," *New York Times*, January 18, 2007, www.nytimes.com/2007/01/18/sports/football/18waters.html (accessed February 1, 2017).

Chapter 18: Marginalized, Minimalized, Ostracized

1. Luke 17:11–19.

2. Tom Gerencer, "How Much Money Do NFL Players Make?" *Money Nation*, January 5, 2016, http://moneynation.com/how-much-money-do-nfl-players-make (accessed February 1, 2017).

3. Cited in Ann McKee et al., "The Spectrum of Disease in Chronic Traumatic Encephalopathy," *Brain* 136 (January 2013): 43–64.

4. Kurt Badenhausen, "Average MLB Player Salary Nearly Double NFL's, But Still Trails NBA's," *Forbes*, January 23, 2015, www.forbes.com/sites/kurtbadenhausen/2015/01/23/average-mlb-salary-nearly-double-nfls-but-trails-nba-players/#6f38440d2d5d (accessed February 1, 2017).

5. Pablo S. Torre, "How (and Why) Athletes Go Broke," *Sports Illustrated*, March 23, 2009, www.si.com/vault/2009/03/23/105789480/how-and-why-athletes-go-broke (accessed February 1, 2017).

Chapter 20: Finding Life in the Wilderness

1. Mark 4:1–20.

2. Romans 12:2.

3. David C. Viano, Ira R. Casson, and Elliot J. Pellman, "Concussion in Professional Football: Biomechanics of the Struck Player—Part 14," *Neurosurgery* 61.2 (August 2007): 313–28, www.researchgate.net/publication/6077137_Concussion_in_profession_football_Biomechanics_of_the_struck_player_-_Part_14 (accessed February 1, 2017).

4. David C. Viano et al., "Concussion in Professional Football: Animal Model of Brain Injury—Part 15," *Neurosurgery* 64.6 (June 2009): 1162–73, www.researchgate.net/publication/26258654_Concussion_in_professional_football_Animal_model_of_brain_injury___Part_15 (accessed February 1, 2017).

5. Bennet I. Omalu et al., "Chronic Traumatic Encephalopathy (CTE) in a National Football League Player: Case Report and Emerging Medicolegal Practice Questions," *Journal of Forensic Nursing* 6.1 (Spring 2010): 40–46, http://onlinelibrary.wiley.com/doi/10.1111/j.1939-3938.2009.01064.x/abstract (accessed February 1, 2017).

6. Jeanne Marie Laskas, "Game Brain: Bennet Omalu, Concussions, and the NFL: How One Doctor Changed Football Forever," *GQ*, September 14, 2009, www.gq.com/story/nfl-players-brain-dementia-study-memory-concussions (accessed February 1, 2017).

Chapter 21: Omalu Goes Hollywood

1. Bennet I. Omalu et al., "Chronic Traumatic Encephalopathy in a Professional American Wrestler," *Journal of Forensic Nursing* 6.3 (Fall 2010): 130–36, http://muchnick.net/omalu_journal_article.pdf (accessed February 1, 2017).

2. Bennet I. Omalu et al., "Chronic Traumatic Encephalopathy, Suicides and Parasuicides in Professional American Athletes: The Role of the Forensic Pathologist," *American Journal of Forensic Medicine and Pathology* 31.2 (June 2010): 130–32, www.protectthebrain.org/documents/CTE_Suicides-and-Parasuicides_Orange-Journal_2009.pdf (accessed February 1, 2017).

3. Bennet I. Omalu et al., "Chronic Traumatic Encephalopathy in an Iraqi War Veteran with Posttraumatic Stress Disorder Who Committed Suicide," *Neurosurgical Focus* 31.5 (November 2011): E3, www.researchgate.net/publication/51761867_Chronic_traumatic_encephalopathy_in_an_Iraqi_war_veteran_with_posttraumatic_stress_disorder_who_committed_suicide (accessed February 1, 2017).

4. Bennet I. Omalu et al., "Emerging Histomorphologic Phenotypes of Chronic Traumatic Encephalopathy in American Athletes," *Neurosurgery* 69.1 (July 2011): 173–83, www.researchgate.net/publication/50227449_Emerging _Histomorphologic_Phenotypes_of_Chronic_Traumatic_Encephalopathy_in _American_Athletes (accessed February 1, 2017).

Chapter 22: *Concussion*

1. Luke 1:38.
2. Matthew 17:20–21.

Afterword: I Bet My Medical License That O. J. Simpson Has CTE

1. Romans 12:2.
2. Matthew 11:19.
3. 1 John 4:7.

Index

Index